TH_
DIABETIC
BRAIN
in Alzheimer's Disease

HOW INSULIN RESISTANCE IN TYPE 2 DIABETES AND
"TYPE 3 DIABETES" TRIGGERS YOUR RISK FOR ALZHEIMER'S AND
HOW YOU CAN PROTECT YOUR BRAIN

RALPH SANCHEZ, MTCM, CNS

The Diabetic Brain in Alzheimer's Disease

How Insulin Resistance in Type 2 Diabetes and "Type 3 Diabetes"
Triggers Your Risk for Alzheimer's and How You Can Protect Your Brain

Ralph Sanchez, MTCM, CNS

Published by: BrainDefend LLC

ISBN: 978-1-7326687-0-6

Disclaimer: The information and ideas in this book are for educational purposes only. This book is not intended to be a substitute for consulting with an appropriate health care provider. Any changes or additions to your medical care should be discussed with your physician. The author and publisher disclaim any liability arising directly or indirectly from this book.

Two FREE Bonuses

Dear Reader,

Two bonus gifts are included with your purchase of *The Diabetic Brain in Alzheimer's Disease.*

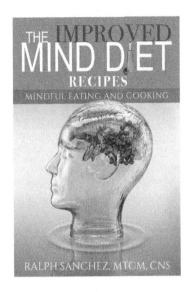

Bonus #1: A week's worth of mind saving recipes from my second book: *The Improved MIND Diet*

Bonus #2: Chapter one from: *The Improved MIND Diet*

Chapter one of *The Improved MIND Diet* details the origin of this powerful dietary plan, and why key food choices can substantially optimize cognitive function and provide crucial protection for your brain against the onset of Alzheimer's disease and dementia as you age.

The Improved MIND Diet recipes are aligned with the primary message detailed in the book—choose and cook your foods wisely, and your brain will benefit greatly for the rest of your life.

To access your bonuses, please type this URL into your web browser's address bar:

ImprovedMindDietBonus.com

Thank you and bon appétit!

*"To heal is to touch with love
that which we previously
touched with fear."*

~Stephen Levine

Contents

Introduction

The twentieth and twenty-first centuries have witnessed a remarkable transformation in the causes of human morbidity and mortality. The industrialization of the economies and food supplies of developed nations, and their associated lifestyle changes, have come at the cost of an increased global burden of metabolic syndrome, type 2 diabetes and cardiovascular disease.(1)

In addition, the projected worldwide incidence of late-onset Alzheimer's disease is projected to increase at an alarming rate and to almost triple by 2050 (2010-2050). One in ten Americans will be diagnosed with Alzheimer's after the age of 65 and that increases to three in ten individuals after the age of 85.

To compound this projected global crisis, the quest for pharmaceutical solutions has been wholly unsuccessful. An analysis of the outcomes of Alzheimer's drug trials conducted between 2002 to 2012 concluded that a staggering 99.6 percent had failed.(2) Nothing has changed since.

Approved pharmacological treatments for late-onset Alzheimer's disease (LOAD), such as cholinesterase inhibitors and NMDA receptor antagonists may provide symptomatic relief and temporarily slow cognitive decline, but do not halt the progression of the disease process—hence these medications are not long-term solutions or curative.

Most clinical trials targeting Alzheimer's disease have aimed to modify primary aspects of the disease process, such as amyloid protein processing and accumulation (associated with amyloid plaque formation), once Alzheimer's has progressed to a more advanced stage. The few trials that have targeted a prodromal and earlier stage of Alzheimer's, mild cognitive impairment, have also failed to demonstrate any significant disease modifying benefit.

Additionally, the drug intervention focus on a singular disease pathway, such as the amyloid pathway, may fail to address a very complex and multifactorial disease process. The emphasis on amyloid pathology, particularly at a later stage of the disease process, is too little and too late. There are many disease mechanisms that converge and promote the expression of Alzheimer's disease in an aging individual.

In chapter five, I detail which type of amyloid protein is the most damaging to the integrity of our cognitive function and is linked to the very earliest stages of LOAD that may precede the diagnosis of dementia by decades.(3)

In fact, the most toxic form of amyloid protein aggregation precipitates LOAD long before the disease process is noticeable in a person, and it is but one component in an interrelated tangle of metabolic, biochemical and hormonal pathways that converge in the pathogenesis of LOAD.

Fortunately, a transformational paradigm shift in the search for a solution to Alzheimer's disease that is centered on risk reduction, and early detection and intervention is now gaining momentum as a viable model for the mitigation of the Alzheimer's pandemic.

Nonetheless, many individuals are only marginally aware of their risk for LOAD, or hardly give a thought to the possibility of their elder years relegated to a life of prescription medications and the eventuality of being placed in an assisted living center—even worse, a center that specializes in caring for those with dementia. Do you ever give that possible aging life scenario for yourself a second thought?

A slogan, "Don't wait to be diagnosed," that I was inspired to use for a Alzheimer's nutrition video training series came to mind recently because it is what so many of us do. We hope for the best and shove the concerns aside until we are diagnosed with an age-related disease such as type 2 diabetes and cardiovascular disease—two of the prime risk factors that increase your risk for late-onset Alzheimer's disease.

If we are confronted later in life by a reality check that type 2 diabetes, or cardiovascular disease is upon us, the integrity of our cognitive function may be already be teetering on the edge of a precipice. How?

Type 2 diabetes, cardiovascular disease and LOAD are increasing viewed as interconnected diseases and the genetic, molecular, biochemical, and metabolic links that are shared by these disorders are now abundantly illustrated in the research literature.

These interrelated disease processes may often progress simultaneously over many years and in many cases they are undiagnosed and unrecognized early in life as potential risk factors for dementia later in life. This is the central theme and rationale for *The Diabetic Brain in Alzheimer's Disease.*

Additionally, women are at increased risk and their heightened susceptibility to Alzheimer's is due in part to midlife metabolic and hormonal alterations that predisposes their brain to metabolic energy deficits and an energy crisis as they age. This presents a priceless window of opportunity for an early detection and intervention strategy of an Alzheimer's related disease process before the irreversible diagnosis of dementia.

Enlightened physicians and clinics around the globe are instituting programs and protocols that are geared toward the evaluation and treatment of cognitive impairment before it progresses to a dementia. Large trials conducted in Europe have shown remarkable stabilization of cognitive decline and early stage Alzheimer's disease with a host of protocols that include dietary and lifestyle interventions, and the monitoring of biomarkers.

The proverbial ounce of prevention long espoused for preventable age-related diseases is now regarded as an enlightened and practical answer to the escalating incidence of LOAD. While there is no cure available for Alzheimer's, it may be a preventable disorder in many cases. If you understand your modifiable risk factors and cooperatively implement a comprehensive and proactive plan for risk reduction, your cognitive skills will likely remain intact.

It is my sincere intention to inspire a proactive approach to preserving your cognitive function—especially if you are at midlife or older. The very same concern for my own risk for dementia inspired my journey to save my brain and I was gratefully blessed with the foundation of Functional Medicine to light the path on how to do so. The rest of the My Story follows in chapter one.

Key Takeaways

- How and why type 2 diabetes and cardiovascular disease increases your risk for late-onset Alzheimer's disease (LOAD).
- Why elevated blood sugar and AGEs (advanced glycation end-products) are toxic to your vascular system and your brain, and how they increase your risk for LOAD.
- How chronic inflammation and oxidative stress mechanisms are central to the development and progression of LOAD.
- Why a deficit in brain energy metabolism leads to a critical energy crisis that increases your risk for LOAD as you age.
- Why your brain gradually loses the capacity to burn glucose as you age and how that increases your risk for LOAD.
- Why women with lower estrogen levels are hypo-metabolic and how this increases their risk for LOAD.
- How a vital energy source (ketones) derived primarily from fat can save your brain from Alzheimer's as you age.
- What is "type 3 diabetes" and brain insulin resistance are and how they're connected to LOAD.
- How the awareness of your specific genetic predisposition to LOAD can reduce your risk for dementia as you age.
- How to evaluate and reduce your risk for the pathological changes that occur in LOAD twenty to thirty years before a diagnosis of dementia.
- How to proactively reduce your risk for Alzheimer's through a personalized health care approach as you age.

Personalized, Precision, Functional and Lifestyle Medicine—what do they all represent?

A note about personalized medicine—a term I use throughout this book. My intention in doing so is to emphasize that an individualized and patient-centered approach to a person's unique set of health-related problems and concerns can best address the health and wellness of an individual—particularly as they age.

Nonetheless, a little history and context is important. The concept of a personalized medicine approach as a clinical healthcare paradigm sprang from the vast information garnered from The Humane Genome Project, which in turn sparked the emerging field of genomic medicine.

Leveraging genetic profiles (genotypes) in the evaluation of risk for a disease process, and the tailoring of interventions for prevention and treatment of diseases evolved into a clinical practice known as personalized medicine.

While the roots of personalized medicine were based on the assessment of an individual's genetic signatures, it has since evolved into more comprehensive science-based approach to an individual's health care through the assessment and analysis of a host of genetic, biochemical, metabolic, and hormonal biomarkers. The reference to precision medicine is often used to denote the same concept and practice. While the two terms are used interchangeably, there is separation of the two terms in the medical community.

The incorporation of a more robust set of biological markers (biomarkers), apart from genetic profiles in the evaluation of their current and future risks to their health, and the individualized medical interventions that may be required to prevent or arrest a disease process has characterized a precision medicine approach.

I also introduce the term "functional medicine", in Chapter 1. Personalized, precision and functional medicine practitioners rely on a similar set of biomarker data derived from diagnostic and functional assessment resources.

However, while the personalized-precision medicine physician may lean toward pharmaceuticals in the clinical management of a case, functional medicine practitioners rely primarily on nutraceuticals, along with dietary and lifestyle based interventions. The importance and emphasis of lifestyle modifications in the management of chronic health conditions had led to yet another clinical model termed: Lifestyle Medicine.

Lifestyle medicine describes the integration of lifestyle interventions such as diet, exercise and stress management, to prevent and treat lifestyle-related diseases such as osteoporosis, type 2 diabetes and cardiovascular disease. Lifestyle medicine may stand alone as an approach to these age-related diseases, or be integrated into the construct of a personalized, precision, or functional medicine framework.

Not to be overlooked in this brief overview of a personalized healthcare approaches are the medical arts and healing traditions that have centuries of empirical evidence in the concept and practice of mind-body medicine. Traditional Chinese medicine (TCM) and Ayurvedic medicine have provided meditation techniques, herbal medicine and acupuncture which have all shown in research studies to benefit aging-related diseases that includes dementia and late-onset Alzheimer's disease. The focus on the whole person, and patient-centered approach is fundamental in the practice of these traditional medical systems.

Regardless of the label, choose your healthcare provider wisely. Are they taking the time to know your personal and family history? Are they fully integrating social, emotional and spiritual factors into their evaluation of what has led to your illness? Are you an active partner in that process? Intrinsically, personalization or individualization of an approach to your health care has many moving parts, and regardless of the method, or the practitioner, one size certainly does not fit all.

Chapter 1

My Story

Alzheimer's. The word alone is enough to conjure up fear and images of lost memories, lost families, lost lives. It's a disease that has no cure and a perception of a regrettable end to a beautiful life. The thought of losing one's memories, their *history*, is often far worse than the prospect of losing one's life. Perhaps for this reason, we push the fear away and *hope* it doesn't befall us or our loved ones.

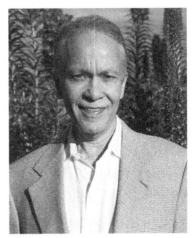

Ralph Sanchez

While the word itself can cause an individual to focus on the tragedy of losing one's mind, it is also a harbinger of folly: a cure. This would be tantamount to claiming there is a true and verifiable cure for any of the chronic degenerative diseases associated with aging. It is merely a fool's gold of expectation, a desperate grasp at slipping around nature. Perhaps someday science will provide an answer for those afflicted with the misfortune of Alzheimer's disease. However, to truly and honestly confront and debilitate Alzheimer's now is to understand that it based solely on *early assessment, intervention, and prevention strategies.*

The lives we live and the choices we make, each and every one, shape us. They shape us while we are children and continue to do so each year of our lives. When we lack appropriate information it becomes difficult to make well-informed decisions. Prevention entails an understanding of the circumstances that can increase the chance of something occurring in the future. Preventing Alzheimer's, adult-onset diabetes, or heart disease entails an awareness of the *risk factors* that are modifiable controls to a path of wellness and vitality, or to one of medication, ill health, and, as in the case of Alzheimer's, the loss of the very cognizance that defines our place in this world.

I'm not here to tell you how you should act or think or what choices to make. What I want you to understand, what I feel is important, is that while there are no guarantees, with greater understanding and information at our disposal, we can choose what our lives will be like ten, twenty, or even fifty years from now. At the time of this writing I am sixty (now seventy), and one of the driving forces in my life is what *I want* my life to be like when I'm eighty, or even, God willing, one hundred. We have the power to control and reduce, to a great extent, our biological future and to minimize, or eliminate, the degenerative diseases associated with aging while maximizing the vast potential of our own lives.

My name is Ralph Sanchez. My road to medicine was neither quick nor of an ordinary path. Many of the details of how I came to this path, this calling to serve through medicine, are better suited for another time and place. Right now I want you to understand *why* I followed this path and why I believe that our road to a long, healthy, and vital life rests within our own power. So, to do this I feel I must share *some* of it with you.

I made my way to the healing arts not solely based on altruistic means; my path to medicine was a spiritual quest. It was inspired by a desire to serve and to become a fully realized person and man. It was also, in part, driven by my own chronic health problems, coupled with my parents' history, that instinctively told me these were issues that the conventional mainstream disease-based and drug-oriented healthcare system could not address. (Perhaps you've felt that, too. That nagging in the back of your mind telling you that your doctor is there to *react* to symptoms rather than get ahead of them.) This model is the cornerstone of medical practice in this country. It's a model that, to put it mildly, is flawed.

During the 1980s, I began experiencing a series of health issues that I eventually attended to in many of my patients. Low energy, chronic colds and flu, mood disorders, allergies, digestive problems, and more. My work at the time was in landscaping, and with all the ignorance and feelings of immortality that are typical of a young man, I endured toxic exposure to pesticides without any regard for my well-being. Unknowingly, the universe had delivered to me the beginnings to my path in medicine. Already fascinated by an alternative model to the very health issues I was dealing with, I sought and found answers in **traditional Chinese medicine** (TCM) and nutritional medicine. I had no idea at the time that my vocation would eventually include these holistic healing traditions.

Indeed, years after experiencing this integrated approach, I would continue my health quest by devoting my life to the study, improvement, and practice of the *complementary health care model*.

The 1980s brought me an intense menu of transformational opportunities. As I looked to my life ahead, I sought to reinvent myself, to find a connection that was lacking. Unhappy with my work and my direction and spurred by this spiritual malaise, I immersed myself in a journey of self-discovery. I'm sure most, if not all, of us have experienced some form of doubt or confusion within our lives, the kind of sensation that we're not doing what we're meant to be doing, not living our passion. I was living a life that wasn't fulfilling, wasn't complete, and a deep, inner sense (some my call it sub-consciousness, others spiritual) was telling me so.

I spent years trying to discover that part of me that was missing, attempting to discover it while I pursued other aspects of my life that I thought were important. After years of a practice of meditation and personal reflection, and the embracement of service as a vehicle of self-realization, I finally found myself in acupuncture school earning my masters degree in traditional Chinese medicine. The doubts, the *ennui*, were gone. I knew what I was meant to do with my life, but this journey had only just begun.

After graduation, I delved into studying a paradigm of medicine, functional medicine, which was inspired by its foremost proponent and educator, Dr. Jeffrey Bland. The essence of functional medicine is to bring together the best of Western medicine, the technology and science, with the complementary medical approach of treating the individual—not the disease. The person is the focus of the healing process, not the illness.

Dr. Bland is a pioneer and internationally recognized leader in functional and nutritional medicine. Co-founder of The Institute for Functional Medicine (www.functionalmedicine.org), Dr. Bland and many other colleagues and distinguished health care professionals have inspired and led the way to a paradigm shift in patient-centered healthcare here in the U.S. and around the world. (Read more about Dr. Bland @: jeffreybland.com.)

In the late 1990s, I bore witness to more serious stage in my mother's cognitive decline. A few years later she was diagnosed with dementia. In looking back, I now understand that there were signs of mild cognitive impairment that was apparent many years before. Just about every other age-related health disorder imaginable occupied the geriatric portion of my practice, but cognitive impairment issues related to neurological disease was not an area that I had much clinical experience with. Nevertheless, with functional medicine as my guidepost for nutritional interventions, I was able to stabilize and slow mom's slide until she could no longer manage taking care of herself.

My mother's mental deterioration brought home once again that my genetic and environmental risk factors put me at tremendous risk to eventually develop the same health disorders that my parents had endured. My mother's and father's health history of cardiometabolic disease—dad died of heart disease in 1979, were powerful reminders that my family history posed a potential and significant genetic risk not only for heart disease, but for neurological disease as well.

By this time I had taken control of chronic inflammation and oxidative stress factors that can elevate risk for heart disease and Alzheimer's, or so I thought. I had instituted an optimal lifestyle and diet, but years later I came to the shocking realization that a chronic urinary tract obstruction that escalated into an acute renal crisis had propelled me into a cluster of cardiometabolic complications, the metabolic syndrome. I was now faced with the stark reality that I had elevated my risk for the very diseases I was dead set on preventing as I aged. A much larger challenge lay ahead of me.

I was now in greater jeopardy of following in my father or mother's footsteps. The cardiovascular disease that brought a premature end to my father's life and the cerebrovascular disease and dementia that led to my mother's passing were potentially in my future as I aged if I did not exercise careful vigilance over the course of my health that was severely compromised. Fortunately, my path in health care and the understanding of the root causes to disease patterns and the underlying risk factors that give rise to them empowered with me the opportunity to save my life and my mind from a similar fate as my parents. The quest for an intact brain in my elder years continues to this very day.

At the time of my mother's cognitive deterioration, I had already begun my research into the neurological complexities of Alzheimer's disease. The role of inflammation and oxidative stress in Alzheimer's disease process, and particularly the genetic links to AD, captivated and fueled my desire for a thorough understanding of how it all worked.

I understood a great deal about powerful brain nutrients that could protect, insulate, and even enhance brain function, but I was now uncovering a wealth of medical research about the biochemical mechanics of the Alzheimer's disease process. What causes the characteristic lesions of Alzheimer's disease (AD)? Why are some individuals more susceptible to developing AD? The more information I ascertained, the more I wanted to find. I was compelled to develop an expertise in the cause and effect phenomena of Alzheimer's. Some might consider it a calling.

That was when the seeds for this book were sown.

As a practitioner of complementary medicine and through an insatiable thirst for understanding the etiologies of disease patterns, I developed a tireless discipline for medical research. My mentors in functional medicine, true pioneers in the evolving paradigm of integrative medicine, provided my new passion with the quintessential role models. The very science and research that they spoke to, was the portal for my own research into the underpinnings of the Alzheimer's puzzle.

I spent countless days and late nights gleaning through the national library of medicine and attending medical conferences and symposiums. It became my mantra for discovery and coalescing an understanding of the roots and causes as to why some individuals develop Alzheimer's disease and why others do not. My passion for the research began to take form in **The Alzheimer's Solution** website content (www.TheAlzheimersSolution.com).

The holism of ancient medical traditions, and that of functional medicine, upholds the timeless model of assessing the condition of the entire person rather than focusing on that individual as a disease entity. It is a *patient-centered model* to clinical practice.

In contrast, traditional Western medicine is a *disease-centered* paradigm that inherently focuses on symptomatic treatment and neglects components that may contribute or, at the very least indicate, the underlying factors of the disease process. The patient is not treated as a whole but rather as compartmentalized components of a greater mechanism.

With regard to Alzheimer's disease, the science is dynamic and has advanced considerably over the past fifteen years—yet the promise of a solution to the growing pandemic is misdirected by the research aimed solely at pharmaceutical interventions. The dismal outcomes to date of drug trials stands in stark contrast to the promising approach of large trials that integrate diet, nutrition, lifestyle, social enrichment, exercise, cognitive training and brain exercises, and the tracking of vascular and metabolic biomarkers (multi-domain intervention trials—PreDIVA, FINGER, MAPT, MIND AD).

Early assessment, intervention and prevention strategies that have served as models for reducing the incidence of type 2 diabetes and cardiovascular disease have gradually emerged as a plausible and hopeful approach to reducing the incidence of vascular dementia and late-onset Alzheimer's disease.

The Diabetic Brain connects the dots that link type 2 diabetes and cardiovascular disease to an increased risk for late-onset Alzheimer's disease and my intention in this work is to raise your awareness and inspire you to save your brain and perhaps even your life. Whether for yourself or a loved one, just know that you're taking a significant and empowering step forward. You can take proactive measures to control of the modifiable and assessable risk factors associated with the onset of Alzheimer's disease.

This book is dedicated to my mother, and to all who are concerned about Alzheimer's disease.

Chapter 2

Insulin Resistance in Metabolic Syndrome and Type 2 Diabetes

One of the most crucial developments in the field of Alzheimer's research over the past fifteen years is the discovery that type 2 diabetes (T2D) and metabolic syndrome (MetS), diseases that are characterized by insulin resistance (IR), have a salient role on the integrity of our cognitive function as we age.

IR may not be clinically apparent until prediabetes or MetS is diagnosed. In many cases, individuals with IR are not diagnosed until frank T2D is apparent. By then, the impact of T2D- and MetS-related disease complications on our neurological integrity may be well on its way to a more consequential neurological disorder. How so?

First, individuals with diabetes and MetS have a substantially higher risk for cardiovascular and cerebrovascular disease, which in turn are recognized as major risk factors for Alzheimer's disease and vascular dementia.

In my introduction I cited a growing consensus regarding the time span of **late-onset-Alzheimer's disease (LOAD)**. The course of the Alzheimer's disease process is now regarded as a twenty to thirty year time frame and the earliest stages of LOAD (preclinical stage), begins without any signs or symptoms (asymptomatic).

Please note the acronyms and abbreviations of IR, T2D, MetS, and LOAD will be used frequently throughout the rest of this book.

Late-onset Alzheimer's disease (LOAD): *The majority of Alzheimer's disease cases represent the late-onset form of the disease. The eventual diagnosis of late-onset Alzheimer's disease (LOAD) is typically after age 65 and the incidence increases with age. Genetic, environmental, and lifestyle risk factors may contribute to the onset of the disease.*

Early-onset Alzheimer's disease (EOAD) occurs earlier in life and represents less than 5 percent of all people afflicted with Alzheimer's.

Onset of EOAD occurs between the age of 30 to 60-65 years and early-onset familial Alzheimer's disease (EOFAD) is considered an inherited form of the disease.

One in ten Americans age six-five and older is diagnosed with Alzheimer's dementia. Given the time frame of decades that the Alzheimer's disease process spans, midlife then becomes a pivotal period for individuals with critical risk factors such as diabetes and cardio-cerebrovascular disease.

Before moving on to how T2D and MetS is more deeply connected to the risk for LOAD and vascular dementia, I will briefly describe the nature of IR and how it arises as it is important to distinguish between the insulin resistance associated with T2D and MetS (peripheral insulin resistance) and central (brain) insulin resistance.

A brain-specific insulin resistance will be described in the last section titled "Brain Insulin Resistance: the Underpinnings of Genetic Risk Variants and Beta-Amyloid Protein."

There are several mechanisms underlying the metabolic alterations observed in patients with MetS and T2D; however, insulin resistance is the most accepted and unifying hypothesis.

Insulin is produced in the pancreas and is the main hormone involved in the uptake of glucose into the cell for energy metabolism. Insulin resistance is defined as an *abnormal* biological response to normal concentrations of insulin at the cellular level.

This means that in order to achieve the same action, one needs much higher levels of insulin to support the action of glucose uptake into insulin sensitive cells—liver, heart, skeletal muscle, and adipose (fat) tissue, as these target tissues become *less sensitive* to the insulin stimulus.

As in MetS, the insulin-resistant state in T2D, which often is a sequelae of MetS, is a metabolic disorder that includes the impairment of insulin function and glucose uptake into skeletal muscle for energy metabolism. Insulin-sensitive cells eventually become desensitized to higher levels of circulating insulin (hyperinsulinemia) and a **down-regulation** of the insulin cellular receptor ensues.

> **Down-regulation:** *the term used to describe the loss of insulin receptor activation (phosphorylation) and function in response to insulin.*

A complex set of dysfunctional intracellular signaling pathways result from the insulin receptor resistance phenomena that is integral to the failed uptake of glucose. A simple illustration that depicts normal and loss of insulin receptor sensitivity is in Fig.1 on next page.

So how does all this begin? In practical terms, IR may develop over time as chronic elevations of insulin are induced after meals (postprandial hyperinsulinemia) or snacks that include more than their share of refined carbohydrates and added sugars.

The subsequent blood glucose spikes place a chronic demand for insulin as the body attempts to maintain normal glucose metabolism.

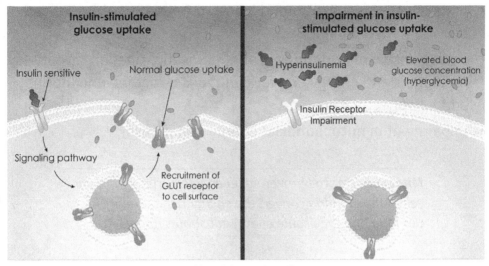

Skeletal muscle cells

Fig. 1

This chronic high blood sugar (hyperglycemia) and hyperinsulinemia cycle sets the stage for T2D in genetically susceptible individuals.

Apart from the diet-induced aspect to IR, a sedentary lifestyle and chronic stress are additional factors that contribute to the potential induction of an insulin-resistant state.

Over time, the ability of the pancreas to maintain a higher demand for insulin is eventually exhausted and hyperinsulinemia morphs into a low insulin secretion state (hypoinsulinemia).

Ultimately, the cellular unresponsiveness to insulin that precipitates IR may initiate the disease process that begins with prediabetes and MetS, and eventually progresses to T2D if preventive dietary and lifestyle measures are not implemented.

Additional molecular and metabolic components that contribute to the genesis of IR include:

- pro-inflammatory molecules (cytokines) produced by visceral adipose tissue (belly fat);

- toxic effect of elevated blood levels of free fatty acids that are derived from belly fat;
- dysregulation of hormones central to insulin function, appetite regulation, and energy and fat metabolism that include leptin and adiponectin, and
- impairment in **mitochondrial** energy metabolism.

Mitochondria: *The proverbial energy factories within our cells. Mitochondria convert the energy-rich nutrients in our food into the usable energy substrates termed ATP.*

These comprise a brief and abbreviated list of mechanisms that contribute to the insulin-resistant state and illustrate just how complex the physiological mechanisms in IR are.

Indeed, the devil is in the details, but the takeaway in this brief overview on the interrelatedness of IR, T2D, and MetS is this:

The predisposing dietary and lifestyle risk factors that drive the insulin-resistant state and the resultant cardiovascular and metabolic (cardiometabolic) disease conditions that gradually unfold have been identified as the very same risk factors for late-onset Alzheimer's disease and vascular dementia.

Lastly, there is a genetic susceptibility that underlies these major age-related diseases of our time. Another link in the chain that connects T2D and LOAD is the *shared genetic susceptibility* between the two disorders.(4) The same is true for cardiovascular disease and LOAD. It is a powerful insight and along with their shared risk factors, it is one that should be at the focal point in evaluating risk for LOAD.(5)

Setting the Stage for the Alzheimer's Disease Pandemic: U.S. and Global Burden of Metabolic Syndrome and Type 2 Diabetes/Cardiovascular Disease

While T2D is generally recognized as an insulin and glucose metabolism disorder by many, the state of IR and conditions of prediabetes and MetS that IR is associated with are not as well understood.

An overview here of their defining features and startling prevalence globally and here in the U.S. will serve to emphasize how it is all connected to the risk for cognitive impairment and dementia as we age.

A clustering of metabolic risk factors commonly termed the metabolic syndrome (MetS) was first designated as syndrome X by Dr. Gerald Reaven in 1988. Also referred to as insulin resistance syndrome, the constellation of metabolic abnormalities put an individual at higher risk for the onset of T2D and cardiovascular disease (CVD).

Current diagnostic guidelines for MetS established by several major organizations that include the International Diabetes Federation (IDF) and the American Heart Association/National Heart, Lung, and Blood Institute is based on the presence of three or more of the following criteria:

- Abdominal obesity (waist circumference >102 cm in men or >88 cm in women).

- Hyperglycemia (elevated fasting glucose ... ≥100 mg/dL or current use of insulin or oral hypoglycemia medication).

- Hypertriglyceridemia (elevated triglycerides ... ≥150 mg/dL.

- Reduced HDL cholesterol <40 mg/dL in men or <50 mg/dL in women).

- Elevated blood pressure (systolic blood pressure/diastolic blood pressure ≥ 130/85 mmHg) or regular use of antihypertensive medication.

This cluster of risk factors associated with MetS increases the risk of cardiovascular events such as coronary heart disease, stroke, and death.(6)

According to data drawn from the National Health and Nutrition Examination Survey (NHANES) from 2003-2012, **approximately 33 percent of American adults met the criteria updated by the American Heart Association and were classified as having MetS in 2011-2012.(7)**

The International Diabetes Federation (IDF) estimates for **prevalence** of MetS is approximately 25 percent worldwide.(8)

Prevalence is a reference for the total number of individuals with a disease or condition that occurs in a specific time period.

Incidence is the rate or number of new cases of the disease in a specific time period.

Overall, the risk of progression to T2D among people with MetS is increased up to five-fold.(9) IDF projections for the prevalence of diabetes globally is expected to increase from 415 million adults to 642 million by 2040.

In the U.S. approximately 9 percent of the population are type 2 diabetics (both diagnosed and undiagnosed) and about 24 percent of those are unaware of their condition.(10)

Prediabetes and diabetes have reached pandemic levels in developed countries. The National Health and Nutrition Examination Survey (NHANES), taken between 2005 and 2008, states that **35 percent of U.S. adults older than twenty years and 50 percent**

of those older than sixty-five years had prediabetes, which corresponds to approximately 79 million adults.(11)

In 2017 the Centers for Disease Control reported that as of 2015, 84.1 million U.S. adults have prediabetes.

By 2030 approximately 472 million adults worldwide are expected to have prediabetes and up to 70 percent of individuals with prediabetes will eventually become diabetics.(11)

T2D and associated cardiovascular disease complications combine to precipitate a host of pathological insults to a vulnerable brain and intensifies the risk for vascular dementia.

The Mayo Clinic Alzheimer's Disease Patient Registry estimated that 80 percent of individuals with Alzheimer's disease have some degree of impaired glucose tolerance or are frank diabetics.(12)

Studies have shown T2D increases the risk for LOAD and vascular dementia by 50 percent, or more, compared with those without T2D.(13) Women have a higher risk than men.(13,14)

These alarming trends on the prevalence of T2D and MetS are linked to the global pandemic of LOAD. The prevalence of vascular dementia and LOAD varies worldwide but is increasing in both developing and developed countries.(15)

Excess visceral fat (belly fat) and obesity is often another potential layer in the prediabetes-T2D continuum and a risk factor that contributes to the pro-inflammatory nature and onset of complications in T2D and CVD (see Fig. 2 on next page). This potent set of disease-related risk factors increases one's vulnerability for the development of vascular dementia and Alzheimer's disease later in life.

Over 60 percent of adults in the U.S. are overweight or obese. One billion persons worldwide are overweight with 300 million deemed clinically obese.(16) However, there are exceptions to obesity as a causative pathway to IR, MetS, and T2D.

Obesity — Chronic Inflammation

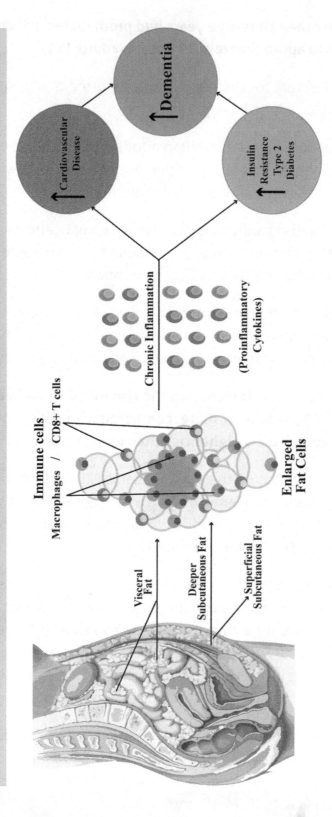

Fig. 2
See description of illustration on next page.

Description of Fig. 2:

Subcutaneous fat is found directly under the skin while visceral fat tissue wraps around the inner organs of the abdominal cavity. Like visceral fat, subcutaneous fat is metabolically active tissue (deep subcutaneous adipose tissue), and both are depots for excess energy intake (calories) and storage in the form of triglycerides.

In obesity, fat cells tend to be enlarged and are a source of free fatty acids derived from triglyceride metabolism that have toxic effects (lipotoxic) on insulin metabolism when elevated. Macrophages and other immune cells are drawn to and associated with enlarged visceral fat cells, which produce more pro-inflamatory cytokines. Excess and enlarged visceral fat tissue is a source of chronic low-grade inflammation (metabolic inflammation) that contributes to the onset of T2D and CVD, and a greater risk for dementia as one ages.

Studies that have examined obese types that are metabolically healthy have shown that up to 25 percent of obese individuals are not IR. They have been designated as metabolically healthy but obese.(17)

Another exception to the obesity link in IR are *persons that are of normal weight and are IR*. Regarded as "metabolically obese normal weight" Individuals (skinny fat body type), they like many overweight or obese types have excess belly fat, elevated blood **lipids** (triglycerides), and are at higher risk for MetS, T2D, and CVD. Body mass index assessments to define obesity in these cases and others will be far off the mark.(18)

> *Lipid disorders: The term describes several conditions in which high concentrations of lipids (fats) exist in the bloodstream. For example, elevated triglycerides, elevated LDL cholesterol, or total cholesterol.*

This metabolically obese-normal weight scenario would likely go without a clinical evaluation of risk which highlights the large number of people with IR and metabolic disease that may go undiagnosed.

With the increased risk that these disease states incur for cognitive impairment in aging, and the spiraling incidence of dementia later in life, a heightened commitment from both the patient and the physician to early assessment and intervention can not be overemphasized.

Hypertension is another common concurrent disease (comorbidity) in T2D and CVD, and it is one of the five qualifying risk markers for MetS.

It is estimated that 75 percent of diabetic adults have hypertension and patients with diabetes and hypertension are twice as likely to have cardiovascular disease complications and stroke events compared to diabetic patients without hypertension.(19,20)

Approximately 85.6 million Americans are living with some form of CVD or the after-effects of stroke.

Midlife cardiovascular risk factors (e.g., T2D, hypertension) vastly increase the likelihood for developing vascular dementia and Alzheimer's disease as one ages.(21)

Impaired blood flow to the brain that is associated with hypertension, stroke, and chronic circulatory system disease precipitates the development of vascular dementia. Additionally, a growing body of evidence now illustrates a causal link between cardiovascular and **cerebrovascular disease**, and the onset of Alzheimer's later in life.

> ***Cerebrovascular disease*** *refers to several medical conditions that affect the blood flow and the circulation to the brain, and the blood vessels that supply it. Narrowing of arteries (atherosclerosis) and hypertension impairs the flow of oxygen and nutrients to the brain and can further restrict cerebral blood flow in the brain that may lead to stroke and transient ischemic attacks (TIAs).*

Fortunately, the emergence of a heart-brain connection concept that illustrates what is good or bad for your heart is also good or bad for your brain is now quickly becoming a model for dementia prevention.

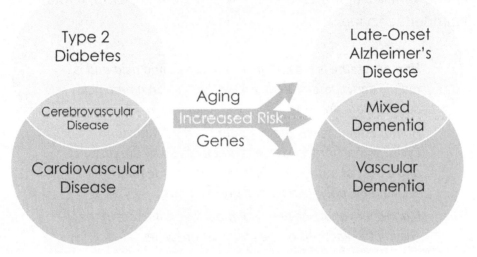

Fig. 3

As noted previously, there are shared genetic susceptibility factors in T2D and LOAD, and the same holds true for CVD and LOAD.

For example, a mutation (genetic variant) of the MTHFR (methylenetetrahydrofolate reductase) gene—C677T, is a common variant in various populations depending on ethnicity and geographical regions. Two copies of the MTHFR C677T variant in an individual (homozygous 677TT), markedly impairs **folate** and homocysteine metabolism, and carriers of the variant have increased risk for stroke, brain shrinkage (atrophy) and neurodegenerative diseases.(23,24,25)

> *In the brain, **folate** and other B vitamins serve a fundamental role in methylation pathways that are essential in the metabolism of neurochemicals (neurotransmitters), the maintenance of nerve sheaths (myelin), DNA methylation and synthesis, and the regulation of homocysteine metabolism.*

Chronic elevations of blood homocysteine is toxic to vascular and brain tissue, and a risk factor in cardio- and cerebrovascular disease, vascular dementia, and LOAD.(5) **Homocysteine** metabolism and its corresponding levels is greatly influenced by genetic variants that include the MTHFR variant C677T, a folate dependent enzyme.

__Homocysteine__ is a sulphur containing amino acid and is mainly derived from dietary methionine—an amino acid derived from protein.

Homocysteine levels are regulated in the "Methylation Cycle" where homocysteine is metabolized by enzymes, and a host of nutrient cofactors that include folate, B12, B6, betaine, polyphenols and antioxidants.

Magnesium and zinc are also important cofactors in the enzymatic reactions of the Methylation Cycle.

Several genetic variants play a critical role in the enzymatic metabolism of homocysteine.

The ApoE4 genetic variant increases the risk of CVD (coronary artery disease) by 40 percent and is the most validated and studied genetic risk factor for LOAD.(15) Carriers of both ApoE4 and MTHFR 677T variants may have an increased vulnerability to the onset of Alzheimer's and vascular dementia.(26,27)

In summary, this rising tide of individuals with cardiometabolic disease will add to the alarming prevalence of Alzheimer's in the years to come and raises serious global concerns with regard to the Alzheimer's pandemic and the societal and economic burden it will impose.

By 2060, almost 25 percent of the total U.S. population will be over sixty-five years of age and the world's population over the age of sixty-five years will more than double by 2050.(18) The oldest old (over eighty-five) is now considered the fastest growing age group in the U.S.(28)

In the U.S., Black/African Americans and Latinos/Hispanics, respectively, have a higher prevalence of Alzheimer's and related dementias over other racial and ethnic groups as they age.(29) A higher prevalence of hypertension, cardio-cerebrovascular disease, T2D, and obesity in blacks and Latinos are considered to be the primary factors. Lower educational achievement and socio-economic factors are considered to be additional determinants of risk.

According to The Centers for Disease Control and Prevention, Latinos are projected to comprise the largest group of older adults in the U.S., and they will have the highest prevalence of Alzheimer's and related dementias among all racial/ethnic groups by 2060.

In all, if we factor the one in ten Americans that will be diagnosed with Alzheimer's disease after age sixty-five and over three in ten after the age of eighty-five, we can easily begin to conceptualize the severity of a crisis that is unfolding.(29)

As emphasized previously in the Introduction, the early diagnosis and adequate treatment of these conditions is paramount to an Alzheimer's and dementia solution. Apart from moderate and short-lived symptomatic treatment, pharmaceutical interventions have failed to deliver any disease modifying benefit.

In contrast, lifestyle, dietary, and nutraceutical interventions have been proposed as promising interventions to modify risk, and for the attendant management of early-stage Alzheimer's disease mechanisms.(30,31,32,33,34)

Clinical evaluation strategies at midlife, if not earlier, that incorporates a set of risk assessments that include biomarkers (biological markers) of cardiometabolic disease, inflammation, and oxidative stress, can provide insights for not only modifying the course of CVD and T2D, it provides a potential risk analysis for vascular dementia, and LOAD.

Biological and neurological markers are measurable indicators of a biological and neurological state, and are utilized in the evaluation of a risk for a disease, the course, prognosis or diagnosis of a disease, and in the management of therapeutic interventions.

Biomarker evidence obtained from bodily fluids (blood, urine, saliva, cerebrospinal fluid), or detection of neuromarkers present in imaging techniques (MRI, PET, CT scans) serve in the assessment of biological and neurologic function and structure.

In late-onset Alzheimer's disease, biochemical, metabolic, and hormonal biomarkers, toxicity testing, genetic testing, and brain scan assessments may facilitate insights into causative factor and risk reduction evaluations, and in the management of disease progression.

The additional concurrent assessment of a person's exposure to environmental toxins, chronic infections, hormonal influences, and genetic risk variants that increase susceptibility to LOAD, can serve as a comprehensive and biomarker-guided approach in the evaluation of current and future risk for vascular dementia and LOAD, and the opportunity for interventions that may vastly reduce the risk for these diseases as one ages.

Chapter 3

Glucose Toxicity, Glycation, and AGEs

The chronic and sustained elevation of peripheral blood sugar (hyperglycemia) is toxic (glucose toxicity) and a damaging force both to the body and brain.

Hyperglycemia precipitates a host of complications associated with diabetes which include eye, kidney, neurological, and vascular disease. Ultimately the degenerative disease processes associated with diabetes and hyperglycemia result in blindness, renal failure, cardio- and cerebrovascular disease, and eventually an untimely death.

The glucotoxic effects of long-term hyperglycemia is classically described in the medical literature as the deleterious effects on pancreatic beta-cell function by chronic elevations of glucose.

The complex metabolic perturbations of glucotoxicity is an ongoing area of research and includes a myriad of mechanisms that are much too complex to describe here. Nevertheless, this metabolic phenomenon is generally accepted as an integral aspect of pancreatic beta-cell dysfunction and the subsequent diminished capacity for secretion of insulin.

In addition, the damaging force of hyperglycemia extends well beyond the glucotoxic effects on pancreatic function. **The toxicity of chronic elevations of blood glucose is mediated by another process termed glycation.**

Glycation reactions (non-enzymatic glycosylation) represent the interaction of glucose with vital structural and functional proteins and lipids (fats) that are integral building blocks of molecules, cells, and tissues of the body.

While glycation reactions are a normal component of metabolism, they escalate as we age due to unhealthy lifestyle and dietary factors and the diminished anti-glycation capacity of our endogenous antioxidant and detoxification defense systems.

Examples of endogenous (internal origin) glycation include the blood test analysis for HbA1c (A1c) that is an indicator of how much glucose is interacting with the hemoglobin protein in red blood cells.

A1c is routinely included in the evaluation of blood sugar control and the risk for T2D. Chronic elevations of blood glucose leads to glycation reactions and it is reflected in the higher percentage of A1c.

An A1c of 5.7 to 6.4 percent is one of the three evaluation criteria utilized in the diagnosis or risk assessment for **prediabetes** that may precede a possible conversion to diabetes.

Prediabetes: The three diagnostic or risk assessment criteria are:
1. blood glucose concentrations of 100 to 125 mg/dl
2. Hemoglobin A1c range (HbA1c) of 5.7 to 6.4%
3. Oral GLucose Tolerance Test result of 140 mg/dl – 199 mg/dl

---

Fructosamine and glycated albumin are additional measures of protein glycation reactions and blood glucose control, and in some cases may be more reliable evaluations over A1c.

Increased glycation reactions that are represented by these biomarkers are indicators of oxidative and pro-inflammatory AGEing mechanisms (more on AGEs below) that are hallmarks of the biological damage that glycation triggers.

Lipid glycation is another element in the glucose-mediated glycation reactions that is in part represented in the damage (**lipid peroxidation**) to cellular membranes (see Fig. 8—page 52) and the lipid constituent of **LDL** and **HDL** lipoprotein particles.

Lipid peroxidation: *Refers to the oxidation of lipids. Lipid peroxidation, and the oxidative damage it represents, has been identified as central to disease processes including cardiovascular disease and Alzheimer's disease.(35)*

---

*LDL stands for low-density lipoproteins and **HDL** stands for high-density lipoproteins. LDL and HDL lipoprotein particles are commonly referred to as LDL and HDL cholesterol due to their major role in the transport and metabolism of cholesterol.*

LDL and HDL lipoproteins are composed of lipid and protein. Varying proportions of cholesterol, triglyceride and phospholipids comprise the lipid component of LDL and HDL lipoprotein particles. These lipids are highly vulnerable to the damage imposed by chronic inflammation and oxidative stress.

Examples of lipid peroxidation biomarkers that may represent these glycation-oxidation pathways (glycoxidation), include oxysterols—derivatives of cholesterol oxidation—and 4-hydroxynonenal (4-HNE). Oxysterols are well know to contribute to many chronic diseases that include CVD and Alzheimer's disease.(35)

4-HNE oxidation of cellular membrane lipids (polyunsaturated fatty acids) is found at increased concentrations in Alzheimer's disease patients, and is linked to amyloid protein aggregation and the disease progression of Alzheimer's.(36)

If unchecked, glycation pathways lead to more advanced metabolic end products referred to as advanced glycation end products (AGEs) and advanced lipoxidation end products (ALEs). AGEs are derived from the glycation of proteins and ALEs are derived from the glycation of lipids (fats). These pathways are illustrated in Fig. 4 (next page) and are detailed in the section on the right half of the illustration.

AGEs and ALEs are toxic compounds (glycotoxins) that can be both produced endogenously—from the toxic interaction of glucose with proteins and fats as described above, and they are also derived from exogenous sources. Diet and tobacco smoke are exogenous sources of AGEs.

The diet end of AGEs and ALEs will be covered a bit further down and needles to say that the toxic compounds in tobacco smoke are a well-known risk for numerous diseases, including Alzheimer's.

Gycation products in tobacco are generated in the curing process and are also termed glycotoxins. These tobacco-derived glycotoxins are precursors to AGEs and eventually form AGEs once they are inhaled. Second hand smoke is a considerable source of glycotoxins.

Glycation reactions and AGE/ALE formation further includes damage and modification of DNA and represents another significant layer to the biological aging process, the risk for disease, and the potential alteration to an individual's genomic stability that is marked by the integrity of DNA maintenance and repair mechanisms.(37)

Biomarker screening and early intervention strategies of these disease processes are paramount. The glycation process may be reversible and represents an early stage event whereas the formation of AGEs and ALEs are not easily reversed.

Both AGEs and ALEs mediate oxidative stress and pro-inflammatory processes that are largely responsible for the long-term related complications associated with the diabetes and cardiovascular

Endogenous Glycation and Formation of Advanced End-Products (AGEs)

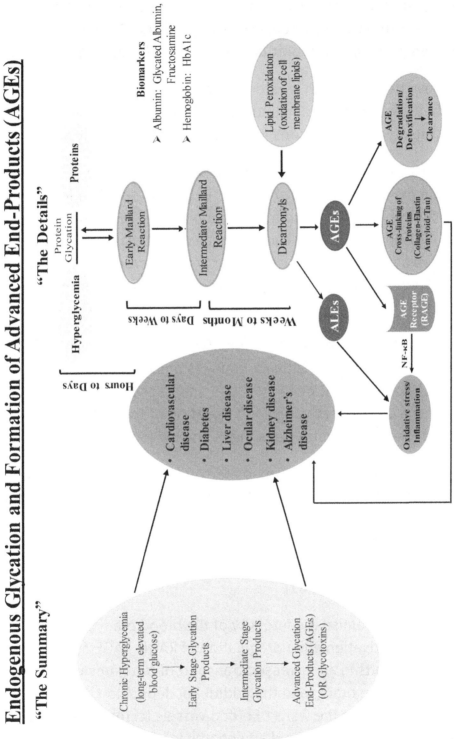

Fig. 4

disease, and AGEs and ALEs are now connected to the onset and progression of neurological diseases that include Alzheimer's, Parkinson's, and amyotrophic lateral sclerosis (ALS).(38)

AGEs have been found in greater concentration in the brains of diabetic patients and amyloid and tau protein in the brain is subject to glycation reactions just as proteins in the body are.

Protein glycation of amyloid and tau protein are molecular constituents in the pathology of Alzheimer's disease. In addition, the toxic effect of AGEs through activation of the receptor for AGE (RAGE) sets in motion a cascade of mechanisms that results in the increased and abnormal processing of amyloid precursor protein and tau protein, and a more neurotoxic beta-amyloid protein. (38,39,40)

Amyloid and tau protein, in the form of aggregates of misfolded proteins, constitute the hallmark brain lesions of beta-amyloid plaque and neurofibrillary tangles that are associated with Alzheimer's disease pathology and glycation of these proteins promotes their aggregation (see Fig. 5 on next page).

Adding injury to insult, RAGE-mediated amyloid precursor protein processing leads to beta-amyloid peptide accumulation, and in turn these amyloid peptides bind to RAGE on microglia (immune cells of central nervous system) to further initiate the pro-inflammatory and oxidative stress pathways that mark the disease progression in Alzheimer's disease.(40, 41)

AGEs also compromise the integrity of the blood brain barrier (BBB) through the activation and upregulation of RAGE. RAGE activation at the BBB results in an increased transport of beta-amyloid from the body into the brain, and the additional deposition of beta-amyloid peptides in the walls of blood vessels (cerebral amyloid angiopathy). Cerebral amyloid angiopathy inhibits blood flow and increases the risk for stroke, brain atrophy, and dementia.

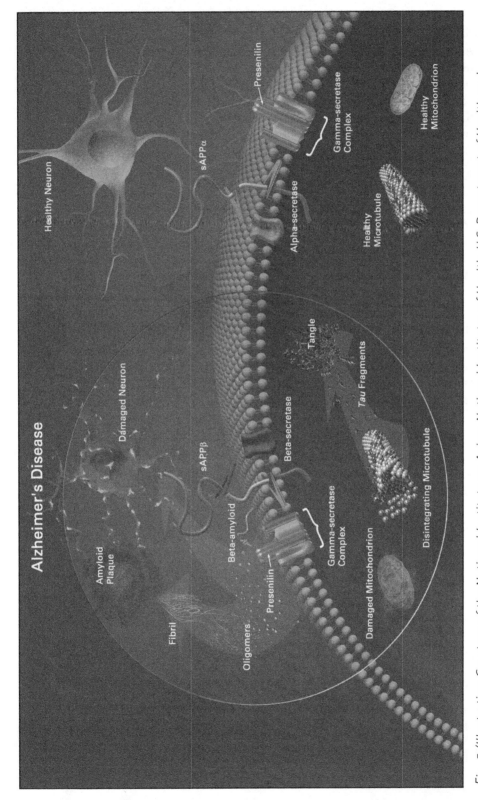

Fig. 5 (Illustration Courtesy of the National Institute on Aging, National Institutes of Health, U.S. Department of Health and Human Services) – See description of illustration on next page.

Description of Fig.5:

The illustration on the preceding page depicts the two major hypotheses associated with Alzheimer's disease—the amyloid hypothesis and the tau hypothesis. Abnormal amyloid precursor protein and tau protein processing results in the two major pathological hallmarks associated with Alzheimer's disease: amyloid plaque and neurofibrillary tangles (NFTs). Note the circled portion of illustration.

The processing of amyloid precursor protein by beta-secretase and gamma-secretase enzymes occurs at the locus of the cellular membrane of the neuron and produces peptide fragments

Beta-amyloid peptides (chains of amino acids) assemble into oligomers and further accumulate into amyloid fibrils which deposit into amyloid plaque. The soluble beta-amyloid peptide aggregates are now linked to the degeneration and loss of synaptic function that occur in the earliest stages (preclinical) of Alzheimer's disease.

Tau proteins interact with other microtubule-associated proteins to promote and stabilize assembly of microtubules that function in part as a structural support skeleton to neuronal dendrites and axons.

Neuronal microtubules provide structure and form to the cell and serve as dynamic conduits for functional materials, organelles, and nutrients that are vital to neuroplasticity (see Fig.14).

Under neuropathological conditions, abnormal tau processing (hyperphosphorylation) destabilizes the microtubule structure and leads to the aggregation of misfolded proteins (neurofibrillary tangles).

Soluble oligomeric tau proteins and neurofibrillary tangles play a central role in the neurodegeneration characteristic of Alzheimer's disease and subsequent cell death.

An additional and important illustration of what occurs in the glycation process is the chemical reaction between carbohydrates and amino acids, and the oxidation of fats in foods cooked at higher temperatures. This chemical reaction, known as the Maillard reaction, describes a culinary phenomena that many foodies love to create by browning foods to enhance flavor and appearance.

Animal derived foods are another significant source of AGEs and cooking AGE-rich foods at a high temperature ultimately results in a host of toxic compounds that include the generation of new dietary AGEs and ALEs (see Fig. 6 on next page).

Dietary Advanced Glycation Endproducts and the Maillard Reaction in Food

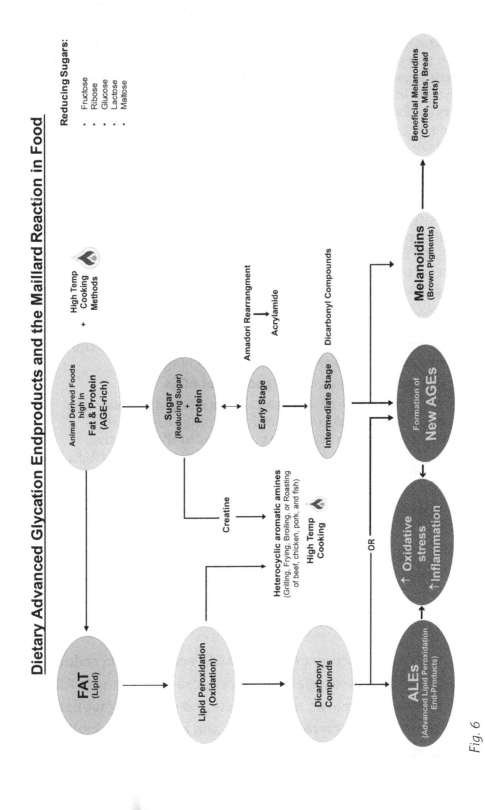

Fig. 6
See description of illustration on next page.

Description of Fig. 6:

The illustration on the preceding page is a depiction of the Maillard Reaction that occurs with higher temperature cooking of foods rich in dietary advanced glycation end-products (dAGEs). The actual formation of intermediate compounds and advanced glycation end-products (AGEs) downstream from the initial interaction of proteins with reducing sugars (e.g., fructose, glucose, ribose, lactose, maltose) are complex and not simply a top-to-bottom or linear chemical reaction process.

The oxidation of fats eventually are stirred into the Maillard stew and there are several branches in the reaction processes that subsequently generate a multitude of compounds that are produced and result from various cooking environments (e.g.,grilling vs. boiling), the type of foods that are heat treated (AGE-rich foods), and the reaction pathways that include desirable (aroma, color, flavor) and beneficial (melanoidin) compounds.

Additional compounds, termed food-borne toxicants—acrylamide, heterocyclic aromatic amines (HAAs) and polycyclic aromatic hydrocarbons (PAHs)—are formed during high-temparature and open-flame cooking and are known to be carcinogenic.

Tobacco smoke is also a significant source of AGEs.

The eventual formation of AGEs and advanced lipid peroxidation end products (ALEs) that are by-products of high-temperature cooking of foods high in fat and protein adds to the oxidative damage and endogenous pool of proinfammatory AGEs and ALEs in hyperglycemic individuals, and may accelerate the degenerative mechanisms associated with diabetes, cardiovascular disease and neurological disease.

Increasing evidence links the intake of dietary AGEs and ALEs in foods with the amplification of oxidative stress and pro-inflammatory responses to the onset of MetS and T2D, and the increased risk for dementia and Alzheimer's disease. (41, 42)

Conversely, the restriction of dietary AGEs and ALEs and reducing the AGE/ALE load is associated with a reduced risk for these AGE-related diseases. Moreover, antioxidants and dietary polyphenols (phytochemicals), and certain vitamins and amino acids inhibit AGE formation and protect against AGE/ALE induced inflammation and oxidative stress.(38, 43)

Chapter 4

Inflammation/Oxidative Stress

The induction of pro-inflammatory cascades and oxidative stress by insulin resistance, hyperglycemia, AGEs, and ALEs comprises a set of constitutive factors in the pathogenesis of cardiometabolic disease and the subsequent risk for vascular dementia and Alzheimer's disease.

Chronic inflammation and oxidative stress are highly interrelated processes and are central to the genesis and **pathomechanisms** of numerous chronic health disorders (see Fig. 7 on next page).

Pathomechanism refers to the pathological mechanism by which a pathological condition associated with a disease occurs. The prefix patho-, is derived from the Greek "pathos" meaning "suffering or disease."

The role of oxidative stress and inflammation in several chronic and age-related diseases such as diabetes, metabolic syndrome, hypertension, coronary artery disease, cerebrovascular disease, and Alzheimer's disease is well established. (44)

Oxidative stress and inflammation are key elements and features of such disease processes, so it is important that before continuing on our journey we understand what these terms mean and their role in chronic degenerative disorders.

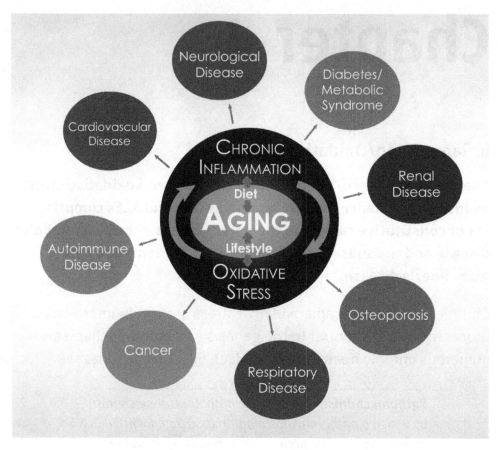

Fig. 7

First, a working definition of "oxidative stress." Oxidative stress is a physiological condition that describes the excessive presence of damaging **free radicals** that counterbalances and overwhelms our endogenous antioxidant defenses.

Oxidative/Nitrative Free Radicals: *Oxidative stress involves reactions mediated by oxygen-containing molecules (reactive oxygen species), while nitrative stress involves reactions mediated by nitrogen-containing molecules (reactive nitrogen species). For example, peroxynitrite (ONOO), a potent free radical, is formed by the reaction of oxygen and nitrogen molecules (superoxide and nitric oxide), and may contribute to the formation of other free radicals.*

The oxidative balance between antioxidants and the oxidants and free radicals that they quench is a key element in optimizing health and buffering against the aging process and some of the degenerative diseases associated with it.

The brain is particularly susceptible to oxidative stress due to three main factors.

The first one is that while the brain represents about 2 percent of the body mass, it consumes approximately 20 percent of the entire oxygen pool. Mitochondrial energy metabolism is a major source of reactive oxygen and nitrogen species that may form **free radicals**.

Free radicals: Free radicals are atoms or groups of atoms with an odd (unpaired) number of electrons, and can be formed when oxygen and/or nitrogen interacts with certain molecules. Once formed, these highly reactive molecules—free radicals—can initiate a chain reaction-like sequence of oxidative/nitrative reactions that are extremely damaging to the cells and tissues with which they interact. Apart from a host of endogenous mechanisms that generate damaging free radicals, environmental exposures to pollution, cigarette smoke, and radiation are among the many external sources that contribute to the cumulative load of highly reactive free radicals that contribute to disease states.

Secondly, the declining levels of natural antioxidant reserves present in the aging brain is a significant risk for cognitive impairment and neurodegeneration.

Lastly, brain tissue is largely made up of fats (approximately 60 percent) that are particularly at risk to damage by oxidative insults mediated by free radicals (see Fig. 8 on next page).

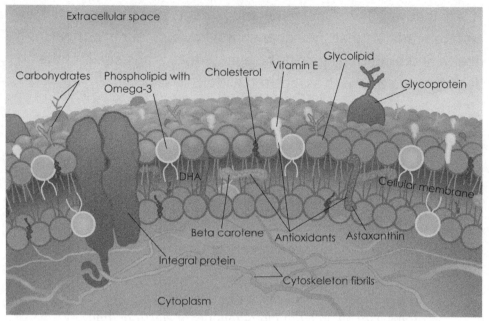

Fig. 8

Description of Fig. 8:

The cell membrane serves as a vital structural and functional element of neurons that is integral to the flow of nutrients, fluids, and signaling molecules into the cell.

Because cellular membranes are largely composed of fats (lipids), they are highly vulnerable to oxidation (peroxidation).

The inner membrane is largely composed of the lipid tail of phospholipid molecules, cholesterol, and fatty acids. The omega-3 fatty acid DHA and antioxidant nutrients, vitamin E and carotenoids, function as essential membrane stabilization and protective compounds.

Proteins embedded in the neuron lipid bilayer function as receptors and transporters.

Carbohydrate chains attached to proteins are termed glycoproteins. Carbohydrates attached to phospholipids are are termed glycolipids. Glycoproteins and glycolipids serve to facilitate signaling mechanisms.

While the lipid structures (cellular membranes) of the brain are at particular risk to oxidative damage (peroxidation), other vital cellular components are just as vulnerable to the assaults initiated by free radicals. DNA and protein structures of the neuron, and their metabolic engines, the mitochondria, are at high risk for oxidative damage. **Such oxidative stress and damage mechanisms are linked to the early stages and onset of Alzheimer's disease. (45,46)**

Oxidative/nitrative stress and chronic inflammation patterns are inseparable. The molecular characteristics of each will invariably perpetuate and exacerbate these interrelated phenomena.

Many exogenous and endogenous vectors of inflammation and oxidative stress cascades are linked to an increased risk of LOAD and vascular dementia as one ages. These pro-inflammatory and oxidative stress mediators that escalate the risk for Alzheimer's and dementia do not emerge over days, weeks, or months; they occur over many years to gradually shift neurological integrity toward neurological disease.

As emphasized previously, the inflammatory pathomechanisms inherent in obesity, T2D, and CVD begin early in life and fuel the smoldering fire of inflammation associated with the increased risk and onset of vascular dementia and LOAD in aging.

Systemic inflammation patterns that are primary to the disease process inherent in obesity, CVD and T2D have been established as principal mechanisms that underlie neuroinflammatory pathways in LOAD.(47)

Chronic cardiometabolic disease and the impaired blood flow to the brain (cerebrovascular disease) further promotes neuroinflammation and oxidative damage, and this vascular dysfunction is a core and early feature in the continuum of the disease process in vascular dementia and Alzheimer's.

In addition, in more vulnerable individuals, inflammation and oxidative toxicity in the brain may be triggered by exposures to neurotoxic elements such as mercury and pesticides.(48,49)

Abnormal aggregates of beta-amyloid and tau protein, chronic infections, mitochondrial dysfunction, a pro-inflammatory diet, and chronic stress (stress hormones) are all drivers of neuroinflammation and oxidative stress in the brain.

These neurotoxic insults stimulate pro-inflammatory pathways that include the recruitment of the resident innate immune cells of the central nervous system—the microglia.

Microglia recruitment and responses to all of the drivers of inflammation detailed in the preceding paragraphs are normal and important housekeeping activities of the microglia, and include the removal of amyloid and tau protein aggregates, pathogens, and damaged and dying neurons through the process of phagocytosis (engulfing and destroying/digesting microbes and cellular debris).

However, the chronic activation (overactivation) of microglia by all of the aforementioned drivers of inflammation and oxidative stress further promotes the production of free radicals and other oxidative cascades.

Microglia overactivation also shifts the normal microglial response, which is neuroprotective, to a pro-inflammatory state with a heightened secretion of pro-inflammatory molecules (cytokines, chemokines).

Microglial overactivation and the "neuroinflammatory axis" in Alzheimer's disease pathology is evidenced and advanced by numerous papers investigating the role of chronic inflammation in Alzheimer's disease.

Furthermore, genetic susceptibility to chronic inflammation adds to the risk of neurodegenerative disease as one ages. Pro-inflammatory genes and genetic mutations linked to inflammation in Alzheimer's driven pathology have also been heavily studied and identified.(50)

Nevertheless, genetic predispositions to inflammation or any number of factors associated with age-related diseases are largely modifiable by diet and lifestyle changes, and an awareness and avoidance of potentially toxic occupational and environmental exposures.

Genes can be turned on in a positive or negative expression. How and why genes are triggered to favorable or unfavorable outcomes in health and disease states is currently an intensely researched field of study referred to as **epigenetics**.

Epigenetics is the study of external modifications to DNA that regulate gene expression without any change to the underlying DNA sequence.

Diet, lifestyle, and exposure to environmental toxins cause epigenetic modifications to DNA that may turn on or turn off certain genes and determines how those genes are expressed (gene expression).

In *The Improved MIND Diet*, I review the powerful role of diet in epigenetic mechanisms. Specific foods can exert a powerful influence on epigenetic modification to our DNA that results in health-promoting and brain saving **gene expression** against chronic inflammation and oxidative stress (Nrf2 activation of antioxidant response element).

Gene expression is the process by which the genetic code of an organism that is inscribed in DNA sequences is copied (transcription) by messenger RNA (mRNA) and is decoded (translation) into a functional and structural proteins by ribosomes that are located in the cell.

Environmental factors such as diet, lifestyle, and toxins induce epigenetic mechanisms that influence gene expression.

Epigenetic therapeutics that include nutrition is a relatively new field of study on how the risk for Alzheimer's and the age-related diseases it is linked to can be modified. It is a research frontier that undoubtedly will help steer the Alzheimer's solution ship toward an early intervention and prevention-centered paradigm.

Chapter 5

Brain Energy Metabolism

Thus far, we have reviewed the correlation of CVD and insulin resistance in T2D and MetS to the heightened risk for vascular dementia and Alzheimer's. Chronic inflammation and oxidative stress bridges many of the interrelated pathways of these diseases.

Another critical feature of insulin resistance patterns in the body and brain is marked by the reduction of energy metabolism as the energy substrate of glucose is unable to be utilized by the the cells energy factories, the mitochondria. Without the fuel to burn a crisis of energy metabolism is set forth.

Peripheral insulin resistance is in part characterized by impaired cellular uptake of glucose and a metabolic perturbation linked to mitochondrial dysfunction.

Similarly, the phenomena of cerebral insulin resistance is linked to reduced rates of glucose metabolism (glucose hypometabolism) and mitochondrial dysfunction that underlies cognitive decline in vulnerable individuals.

The decline in brain energy metabolism distinguished by glucose hypometabolism and and mitochondrial dysfunction are a significant set of related risk factors that are now viewed as early metabolic antecedents that set the stage for the onset of late-onset Azheimer's disease (LOAD). (51)

The brain is an avid glucose consumer, and under normal circumstances the brain's energy demands are provided almost exclusively by glucose metabolism. In this regard, the brain is quite an expensive organ; while accounting for only approximately 2 percent of the body weight, the energy required to maintain brain functions represents approximately 20 percent of an individual's resting metabolism. In fact, the human brain consumes around 100 to 120 grams of glucose per day.

With regard to mediating glucose uptake into the neurons and the role of insulin-stimulated glucose metabolism, the brain has long been regarded as an insulin-insensitive organ. However, there is evidence that key regions of the brain are in part reliant on insulin mediated glucose uptake into brain tissue via insulin stimulated mechanisms.

The details and research are intricate but the takeaway of insulin's role in neuronal glucose metabolism is supported by recent studies.(52)

Thus, when central (brain) insulin signaling is disrupted, glucose metabolism is impaired and neurons do not have enough energy (ATP) to meet their demands.

Over time, the consequent depletion of ATP results in an energy crisis that sets in motion damaging signaling cascades that places mitochondrial function and cell survival at risk.

While insulin fulfills a role in glucose metabolism in the central nervous system, glucose itself is not the sole substrate for energy metabolism in the brain. Recent evidence suggests that lactate serves as an important fuel derived from astrocyte mitochondrial metabolism and may be the primary substrate for energy metabolism in neurons.

Lactate is supplied to neurons from glucose metabolism by astrocytes and it is metabolized from glycogen stores in the astrocyte. The "astrocyte–neuron lactate shuttle" (ANLS) model describes a supplementary pathway for meeting the demands of energy metabolism in the brain.

Lactate (lactic acid) has long regarded as solely a waste product of energy metabolism (anaerobic). However, lactate is now understood to serve as an supplementary substrate to glucose for energy metabolism in the brain, heart, skeletal muscle, and other tissues.

More recent explorations into the synergism between astrocytes and neurons indicate that lactate metabolism is essential to the formation of memory mechanisms and may be a preferred neuronal energy substrate. (53)

Apart from the understanding that lactate metabolism is an important insight into the workings of brain energy metabolism, the ANLS model illustrates the vital role that **astrocytes** serve in the energy flux between the neuron and the astrocyte. This also applies to the metabolism of fats (fatty acids) and ketones.

Astrocytes (star-like cells), also known as astroglia, function in numerous and vital roles in the central nervous system (CNS) that are essential to brain homeostasis. The close interaction between astrocytes and cerebral blood vessels (neurovascular coupling) is a dynamic bridge in the nutritional, metabolic, and protective support astrocytes provide to neurons.

Steps 1 through 3 in the ANLS illustration on the next page exhibits the uptake of glucose from brain capillaries into the astrocyte where it is converted to lactate and subsequently transported into the neuron where it it is taken up into the mitochondria for energy metabolism.

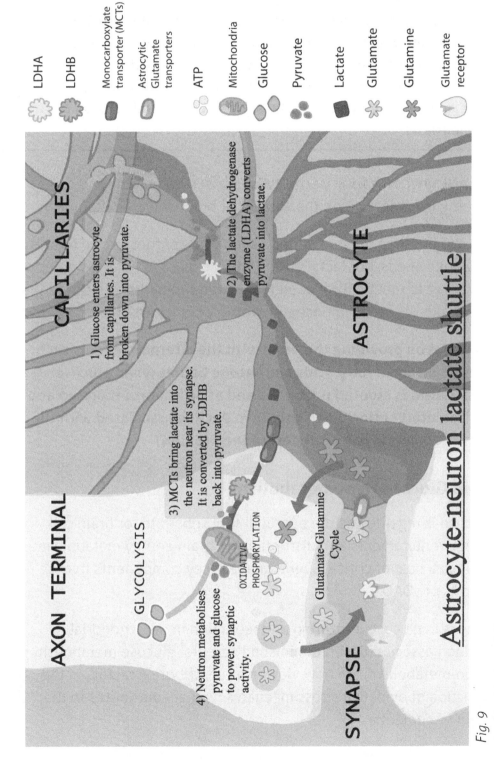

Legend:

- LDHA
- LDHB
- Monocarboxylate transporter (MCTs)
- Astrocytic Glutamate transporters
- ATP
- Mitochondria
- Glucose
- Pyruvate
- Lactate
- Glutamate
- Glutamine
- Glutamate receptor

CAPILLARIES

1) Glucose enters astrocyte from capillaries. It is broken down into pyruvate.

2) The lactate dehydrogenase enzyme (LDHA) converts pyruvate into lactate.

ASTROCYTE

AXON TERMINAL

GLYCOLYSIS

3) MCTs bring lactate into the neuron near its synapse. It is converted by LDHB back into pyruvate.

OXIDATIVE PHOSPHORYLATION

4) Neuron metabolises pyruvate and glucose to power synaptic activity.

Glutamate-Glutamine Cycle

SYNAPSE

Astrocyte-neuron lactate shuttle

Fig. 9
See description of illustration on next page.

Description of Fig. 9:

Astrocyte-neuron metabolic interactions that include lactate and ketone shuttle systems, and the utilization of glucose, lactate, glutamine, and ketones for energy metabolism is critical in powering and maintaining the high energy requirements of synaptic activity (e.g., glutamate-glutamine cycle) and preserving brain energy homeostasis.

The ANLS hypothesis in part serves to assert a complex and ongoing investigation on the subject of brain energy metabolism.

Glucose has long been regarded as the primary fuel for the brain's metabolic needs, but lactate, fats (fatty acids), and ketone bodies also serve to meet neuronal metabolic requirements as stage of life and health disorders impose its own set of circumstances.

The focus on providing the brain with the alternative fuels such as medium chain fatty acids and ketone bodies when glucose metabolism is blunted is now viewed as an important option and clinical intervention when cognitive decline associated with the risk for dementia has been determined.(51,54)

Brain Glucose Hypometabolism

Glucose is regarded as the essential fuel substrate for brain cell energy requirements and disruptions in brain energy metabolism leads to a host of critical events that are key components to the genesis of LOAD.

Deficits in glucose utilization and reduction in mitochondrial function associated with diminished cerebral glucose metabolism (hypo-metabolism) are now viewed as contributing factors in the induction of oxidative stress mechanisms that contributes to the onset of dementia.

Glucose hypo-metabolism, the term used to describe the impaired utilization of glucose in the brain, has been shown in several studies to be a specific correlate to the cognitive dysfunction in the early stages of mild cognitive impairment (MCI), and to the eventual development of LOAD. (55)

Not only do individuals diagnosed with MCI and LOAD have lower rates of brain glucose metabolism, carriers of the ApoE4 gene variant, a prime genetic susceptibility marker for LOAD show a decreased rate of glucose metabolism at a young age—years before any evidence of brain function abnormalities. (55)

A progressive decline in cerebral metabolic rates of glucose (CMRglu) is linked to brain atrophy (shrinkage) and both abnormalities can serve as indicators of the very earliest stage (preclinical) of Alzheimer's disease.

One of the most promising outcomes in the research related to cerebral glucose hypometabolism is the emergence of FDG-PET scans (fludeoxyglucose F 18–positron emission tomography) in the evaluation of patients deemed at higher risk for a progression of MCI to dementia.

The potential for neuroimaging assessments such as PET for the early detection and possible prevention of LOAD is proposed in several studies.(57)

Individuals with the early signs of MCI now have significant neuroimaging tools available through their physician for gauging a potential risk in the development of LOAD.

Previously regulated to clinical studies that sought to standardize analysis and interpretation criteria for clinical applications, PET and Magnetic Resonance Imaging (MRI) are now widely available, and are noninvasive screens that might provide invaluable opportunities to leverage assessment and intervention strategies in the earliest stages of cognitive decline.

Obstacles include cost, patient tolerance, and exposure to radioactive tracers in PET. Nonetheless, neuroimaging screens may provide invaluable insights into and **hippocampal** volume (atrophy), pathology (Abeta, tau protein), and metabolic abnormalities (glucose hypometabolism).

Hippocampus: a seahorse-shaped structure in the brain (medial temporal lobe) that is a key region linked to complex memory and learning mechanisms, spatial navigation, and in the processing of emotions.

Hippocampal volume changes and atrophy rates correlate with the structural and functional degeneration associated with aging and the earliest stages of the Alzheimer's disease process.

As stand-alone assessments, neuroimaging screens are not highly accurate (specificity-sensitivity) due to several variables. Lack of standardization is often pointed out as a rationale for not recommending neuroimaging as a diagnostic screen for Alzheimer's related pathology.

However, when imaging is combined with:

- **cognitive assessments (e.g., GPCOG, MoCA),**

- **evaluation of genetic susceptibility (ApoE4),**

- **inflammation and oxidative stress biomarkers (e.g., pro-inflammatory cytokines, *8-OHdg*), and**

8-OHDg (8-hydroxy-2" deoxyguanosine) is a biomarker of oxidative stress and damage to DNA (oxidized DNA guanine lesions).

- **vascular and metabolic (cardiometabolic) pathology biomarkers,**

a priceless window of opportunity for an integrated evaluation of risk for cognitive decline, and the timely interventions in preclinical Alzheimer's disease (asymptomatic) and mild cognitive impairment (symptomatic), becomes possible.

Brain Energy Metabolism-Ketosis

To recap, the decline in glucose utilization and brain energy metabolism (neuroenergetics) is a primary risk factor in the onset of LOAD. Glucose hypometabolism and mitochondrial dysfunction is increasingly recognized as the earliest set of metabolic aberrations that precedes the more progressive cognitive decline associated with Alzheimer's disease.

Fortunately, the role of fatty acid and ketone energy metabolism has emerged as a rescue intervention to glucose hypometabolism and the brain energy crisis that follows.

Ketones function as a critical substrate to fuel brain energy metabolism when glucose and lactate energy metabolism is blunted.(58)

In conditions that reflect disruptions in the astrocyte-neuron funnel of glucose and lactate metabolism, (recall the astrocyte-neuron lactate shuttle in Fig. 9?): the utilization of alternate metabolic fuels is critical to the maintenance and survival of the brains's cellular stability. This is where ketones enter center stage.

Fats (fatty acids) cross the blood brain barrier (BBB) and contribute to significant mitochondrial metabolism in the brain. Recent experimental research has shown that fatty acids readily cross, or are transported across the BBB and contribute to lactate and ketogenic metabolism in astrocytes.(59,60)

Just as they supply lactate to the neuron for energy metabolism, astrocytes provide ketones (astrocyte ketogenesis) in what has been described as the astrocyte-neuron ketone body shuttle. These neuron-astrocyte metabolic interactions are are not only vital to maintaining the high neurometabolic energy requirements for our brain cells, they are also neuroprotective against cognitive decline and neurological disease.

Recent investigations have shown that fatty acids serve as a viable energy metabolism substrate and that 60 to 80 percent of the brain's mitochondrial fuel can be suppled by ketones—acetoacetate and betahydroxybutyrate that are derived from the metabolism of fatty acids by astrocytes.(61,62,63)

The compensatory shift from glucose metabolism when impaired to the metabolism of medium chain fatty acids and ketones in the brain can support an adaptive response to the reductions in cerebral glucose metabolism associated with the progression of cognitive decline in Alzheimer's.(64)

In the brain, ketone metabolism protects neurons from the toxic effect of beta-amyloid protein and provides neuroprotective benefits through several inhibitory mechanisms on excitotoxicity, inflammation, and oxidative stress. (65,66,67)

Significant mitochondrial benefits are derived from brain ketone metabolism that includes a reduction in mitochondrial oxidative stress and increased glutathione levels as a result of more efficient metabolism (mitochondrial bioenergetics), and an increase in mitochondrial biogenesis—the formation of new mitochondria from pre-existing mitochondria (growth and division).

Caloric restriction and intermittent fasting is also associated with signaling pathways that stimulate mitochondrial biogenesis.(68,69) Both caloric restriction and intermittent fasting interventions can compliment nutritional ketogenesis and provide remarkable benefits for preserving and optimizing cognitive health and longevity.

Endogenous generation of ketones (ketogenesis) is facilitated through dietary therapy—a low carbohydrate/high fat diet (ketogenic) and similar diet therapies, and in states of caloric restriction diet therapy.

In caloric restriction fatty acids derived from body fat tissue is metabolized (lipolysis), and can be utilized for energy metabolism and ketone synthesis.

The metabolic shift from carbohydrate dependent energy metabolism to the mitochondrial oxidation of fatty acids and ketone body synthesis in both ketogenic diets and in caloric restriction is commonly referred to as ketosis (see Fig. 10 on next page).

In ketogenic diet therapy (KDT), a low carbohydrate and high fat diet optimizes the supply of fatty acids to the liver for the synthesis of ketones (nutritional ketogenesis).

Restriction of calories is not the explicit goal in KDT and ultimately, KDT may serve as a more attractive choice for individuals that may struggle with a more restrictive caloric restriction model.

Medium chain triglycerides (MCTs) supplementation has recently exploded in the health market place as an optimal means to enhance nutritional ketogenesis. MCTs are metabolized to medium chain fatty acids (MCFAs).

MCFAs are rapidly absorbed into circulation (portal vein) and transported directly into liver mitochondria for metabolism, while longer chain fatty acids (LCFAs) requirements for intestinal absorption and transport to the liver are more complex (see Fig. 10 on next page).

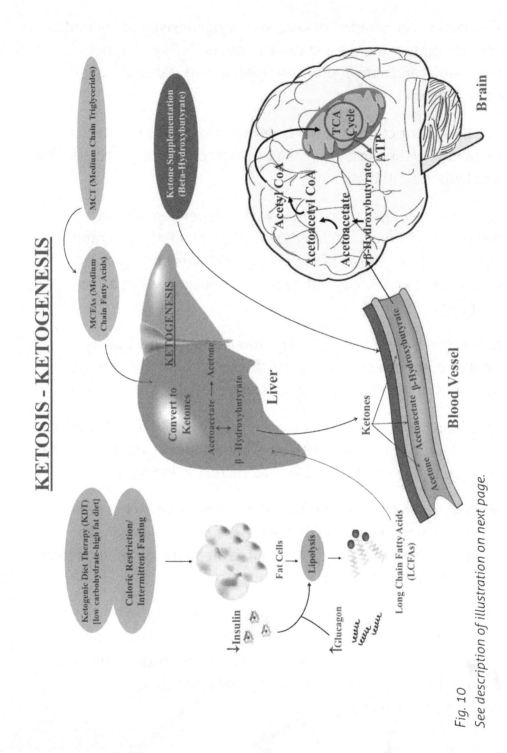

Fig. 10
See description of illustration on next page.

Description of Fig. 10:

The left side of the illustration on the preceding page depicts the mobilization of fatty acids (LCFAs) from fat tissue while the right side of the illustration depicts the metabolism of medium chain fatty acids (MCFAs) derived from the intake of medium chain triglycerides (MCTs). Ketone supplementation (beta-hydroxybutyrate) is another option for elevating serum ketone esters for energy metabolism.

The metabolic state of ketosis derived from ketogenic diets mimics the state of caloric restriction (CR) and fasting, and enables a compensatory shift from a glucose predominant energy metabolism to one that preferentially utilizes ketones for energy metabolism in tissues that are able to metabolize ketones—e.g., brain, heart, and skeletal muscle.

The fatty acid metabolism and generation of ketone bodies (ketones) transpires in the liver and is exported and to support energy metabolism in other tissues. The liver can not utilize ketones for energy metabolism.

In the brain, the availability of ketones for energy metabolism compliments lactate and glucose metabolism. In aging and neurological disease the availability of ketones is critical to energy homeostasis and mitochondrial bioenergetics. Insufficient energy substrates for mitochondrial energy metabolism compromises mitochondrial and neuronal integrity which contributes to the pathomechanistic features associated with the early stages of cognitive decline and neurological disease associated with Alzheimer's disease.

Fatty acid metabolism in the liver and the subsequent production of ketones that are high energy substrates can readily pick up the slack when glucose is unavailable or utilization is inhibited. Hormones (insulin, glucagon) play a role in what amounts to an orchestration of metabolic and endocrine pathways that have evolved to sustain energy metabolism when calories are scarce.

Elevated insulin levels associated with insulin resistance (hyperinsulinemia) inhibit release of fatty acids (lipolysis) from stored fat in the body and caloric restriction is an ideal dietary approach for lowering insulin in hyperinsulinemia.

It is important to distinguish a regulated or preferred generation of ketone bodies from metabolic disorders that involve defects in fatty acid transport and metabolism (inborn errors of metabolism), or pathological states that result in ketoacidosis—a condition of excess serum ketones associated with diabetes and other disorders.

The controlled endogenous synthesis of ketones is prompted by low blood glucose levels that result from low carbohydrate and caloric restriction diets, intermittent fasting, or in prolonged intense exercise that exhausts stored energy (glycogen) reserves. It is a normal, vital, and adaptive response to lack of glucose for energy metabolism.

KDT, caloric restriction (CR), fasting and various types of intermittent fasting (IF), is now utilized to manage obesity, hyperglycemia, and IR in MetS and T2D.

KDT, IF, and CR improves insulin sensitivity and results in dramatic reversal of T2D biomarkers and the disease process. Similar benefits have been demonstrated in the management of cardiovascular disease with CR, fasting, IF, and KDT.

Promising results in human studies suggest that these dietary protocols are effective intervention options in cardiometabolic disease and the risk for dementia. Additionally, in cases where the risk for cerebral glucose metabolism has been determined, or evidence of cognitive decline exists, MCT and ketone supplementation to drive ketone metabolism may be superior neurometabolic rescue interventions.(70,71,72)

Decrements in brain glucose metabolism and mitochondrial function occurs in aging and in the earliest stages (preclinical) of Alzheimer's decades before any neurodegeneration is observed and it is in this critical stage where supplemental support with

MCTs and ketones (betahydroxybutyrate) is proposed to be the most advantageous.(67,73)

Family history provides another crucial insight into brain energy deficits that can she light on the evaluation for the risk of Alzheimer's when it includes a maternal history of the disease versus a paternal history.

Mitochondrial DNA is maternally inherited and mitochondrial defects that contribute to the risk for brain metabolic deficits that include glucose hypometabolism and oxidative stress is seen in adult offspring of mothers with a history of Alzheimer's.(74)

Apart from family history, sex and risk genes are factors that patient and their physician can weigh into a neuroenergetic risk assessment when there is a concern for dementia later in life.

The ApoE4 genetic susceptibility variant is associated with glucose hypometabolism and mitochondrial dysfunction. Ironically, administration of MCTs in patients appears to be more beneficial in noncarriers of the ApoE4 variant. (66,75)

There is, however, evidence of improvement of cognitive function with intake of MCTs and ketone ester supplementation in an ApoE4 positive individual that experienced severe cognitive decline in his 50s. Results of his Mini-Mental State Examination (MMSE) and neuroinmaging assessment (MRI) were consistent with Alzheimer's dementia.(76)

Unfortunately, to date there is a lack of research in the area of ketogenic diet therapy (KDT), or ketone supplementation in ApoE4- positive individuals that would shed more light on the the underlying factors that may explain why there may be an ApoE variant dependent outcome that results from KDT or ketone supplementation.

Preliminary research indicates that insulin signaling and other genetic variants associated with insulin metabolism in the central nervous system as probable factors.

The role of insulin and genetic variants in ketone metabolism notwithanding, sex differences in neuroenergetic deficits that occur in aging is an essential component in the evaluation of risk for cognitive decline and Alzheimer's.

Women are more susceptible to the onset of Alzheimer's as they age and the biological changes that occur at midlife may have profound neurological effects later in life.

In women, estrogen regulates brain and body glucose metabolism and mitochondrial function, and a decline in estrogen in menopause is commensurate to a decline in cerebral glucose metabolism.

A decline in cerebral glucose metabolism in low estrogen states results in a compensatory shift to ketone metabolism that is known to occur in the menopausal transition.

Brain specific ketone metabolism in women at menopause may be at the expense of the all important myelin sheath that surrounds the axon extension of neurons that insulates and enables electrical transmission.

Myelin is approximately 70-80 percent composed of lipids and in susceptible individuals, myelin can be metabolized to provide fatty acids for ketone synthesis. (64,77) **Female ApoE4 carriers with declining estrogen levels appear to be more vulnerable to an earlier age onset of myelin breakdown and the the onset of neurological disease.**

These risk associations are critical components in evaluating Alzheimer's risk in females when factoring in estrogen decline in midlife and the ensuing reductions in glucose metabolism.

In the U.S., the prevalence of LOAD for women sixty-five years of age and older is almost two-fold higher than men. (78)

While KDT and MCT therapy have shown to be promising approaches in boosting cognitive performance in mild cognitive impairment and Alzheimer's disease, the support of ketone and mitochondrial metabolism earlier in life may indeed result in dramatic dividends that optimizes brain bioenergetics, improves cognitive function, and supports healthy brain aging.

Not to be overlooked are potential side effects of nutritional ketosis. The elderly and patients with diabetes and medications should be medically supervised as blood lipids, blood pressure and kidney function, liver function, and body fluid and electrolyte imbalances are common concerns in KDT.

Gastrointestinal (GI) side effects such as nausea, vomiting, diarrhea, and constipation in KDT are usually short-term and more likely when supplementing with MCT products. "Keto-flu" and GI side effects may be minimized or avoided with a gradual introduction of KDT, fluid, electrolyte and fiber intake, and complementary supplementation.

Chapter 6

Brain Insulin Resistance: the Underpinnings of Genetic Risk Variants and Beta-Amyloid Protein

Our journey thus far has described the metabolic mayhem mediated by cardiometabolic disease and the associated patterns of hyperglycemia, insulin resistance, inflammation, and oxidative stress that are linked to the pathogenesis of LOAD.

Ultimately, peripheral insulin resistance and T2D, and the comorbidities of CVD (hypertension, atherosclerosis), puts one at a heightened risk for vascular dementia and type 3 diabetes—a brain specific insulin resistance.

The hypothesis of a "type 3 diabetes" that described the loss of insulin function in the central nervous system was first described in 2005 by a team of researchers that included Dr Suzanne M. de la Monte, a neuropathologist and professor of pathology at Brown Medical School.

This seminal research that linked an "insulin resistance" like pattern in the brain to AD pathology has since been examined and illustrated in numerous research models and papers led by Dr. de la Monte M.D., M.P.H., Suzanne Craft, Ph.D., William L. Klein Ph.D., and other pioneers in the Alzheimer's-cerebral insulin resistance research frontier.

The central insulin resistance criterion provides a framework for an enlightened understanding of the synaptic signaling mechanisms that are at the core of brain plasticity and how the dismantling of these fundamental processes that are vital to cognition underlies the cognitive decline in type 3 diabetes.

The signaling dynamics of insulin and insulin growth factor (IGF) function in the brain is integral to **synaptic plasticity** and subsequently one's cognitive competence.

Synaptic plasticity: *Brain plasticity is the bird's eye view of synaptic plasticity. The cellular and molecular basis of synaptic plasticity is represented in part by receptor mediated signaling mechanisms and cascades integral to synaptic transmission (described in this book) that underlie learning and memory processes.*

On the other hand, the inhibition of insulin's effect on neuroplasticity underlies the disrupted synaptic terrain associated with the neurodegenerative aspects of LOAD and is now described in numerous studies as brain (central) insulin resistance.

Neuroplasticity, also known as brain plasticity, refers to the brain's capacity for adaptive change. Brain plasticity is reflected in the brain's ability to integrate change associated with learning, organize that experience, and form new neural connections and pathways that supports and enables that process.

Plasticity processes occur throughout a person's lifetime—as a young brain grows and develops, as a mature brain integrates new information and learning, or as it recovers from brain trauma (traumatic brain injury).

Insulin and synaptic neurochemicals serve as integral mediators of plasticity mechanisms vital to healthy brain aging throughout one's lifetime.

Insulin binds to receptors at the synapse, a key communication locus between neurons in the brain. Synaptic junctures between neurons is where the cell-to-cell brain circuitry is facilitated (see Fig. 11 on next page).

Insulin is now known to serve as a vital element for synapse maintenance (structure and function) and subsequently for the strength of connections between neurons. (79) This insulin/synaptic axis and the formation of new circuitry in the brain is a key contributor to brain plasticity.

Ultimately, brain insulin and insulin receptor signaling are requisite mechanisms in the maintenance and survival of the synapse.

In contrast, central insulin resistance and its role in LOAD is characterized by the down-regulation of synaptic insulin receptors and the consequent loss of insulin signaling mechanisms.

The diminished function of insulin at these critical junctures is now viewed as representative of the corresponding neuropathological events in the earliest stages of cognitive decline that characterizes the progression of LOAD. (80)

So how do we lose it? What are the root causes in the trail of numerous immune, molecular, and biochemical steps that leads to brain insulin resistance and Alzheimer's disease—the loss of cerebral insulin receptor function and synaptic signaling integrity, and the consequent soundness of our cognitive processing capabilities?

As described earlier, peripheral insulin resistance, hyperglycemia, glycation and advanced glycation end-products, greatly contribute to the vascular pathomechanisms that underly the progression of cardiometabolic disease.

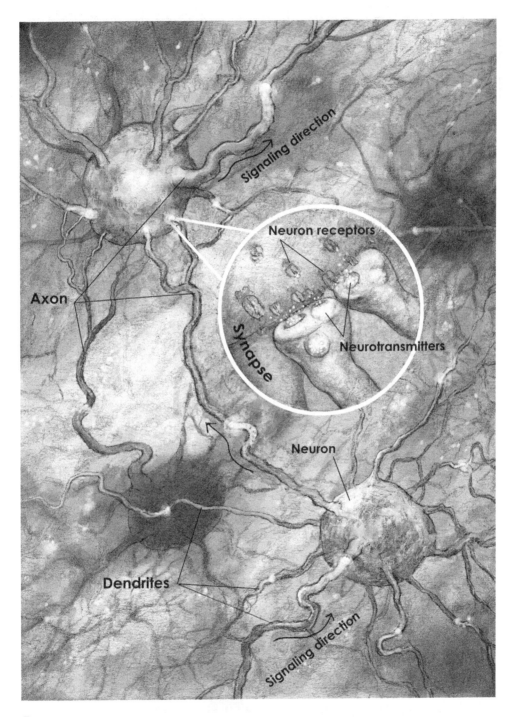

Fig. 11
See description of illustration on next page.

Description of Fig. 11:

Synapses are specialized junctions between neural cells, or neurons. The complex network of neuronal synapses function to transmit electrical and chemical signals from one neuron to a another (synaptic transmission).

Synaptic transmission begins with an electrochemical impulse that travels down the axon and its branches and results in the release of neurochemicals (neurotransmitters) from the presynaptic axon terminal. Neurotransmitters move across the synapse (synaptic cleft) and bind to postsynaptic receptors on dendrites, axons, and on the neuronal cell body.

In turn, peripheral insulin resistance and the associated pro-inflammatory and oxidative stress patterns linked to cardiometabolic disease advance the very same insults into the brain, which significantly increases the risk for vascular dementia and LOAD.

The complications of cardiometabolic disease progresses over years and the overlapping pathological associations between cardiometabolic disease, cerebrovascular disease, and Alzheimer's can span decades before a diagnosis of dementia.

Environmental factors such as diet, lifestyle, and toxins act as triggers to disease expression, and **genetic variants** underlie susceptibility for an individual and the genetically linked triad of T2D, CVD, and LOAD.(81,82) To the point and a favorite quote: *"Genes load the gun and environment pulls the trigger."* (Cynthia M. Bulik Ph.D.)

Genetic variants *that have a certain degree of risk associated with onset of a disease are termed "risk variants". Individuals with the ApoE4 variant have an increased risk of developing late-onset Alzheimer's disease*

Susceptibility Genes

The ApoE4 risk variant is the most validated genetic risk factor for LOAD. However, a broadening pool of risk variants associated with several genes (e.g., BDNF, TREM2, TOMM40, SORL1, PICALM), have been identified in many independent and genome-wide association studies (GWAS) as risk variants in LOAD. The added discoveries in potential risk variants for LOAD has led to the growing understanding that LOAD is a **polygenic** (two or more genes) disorder.

Polygenic *disease results from the effects of the combined action or interaction of multiple genes.*

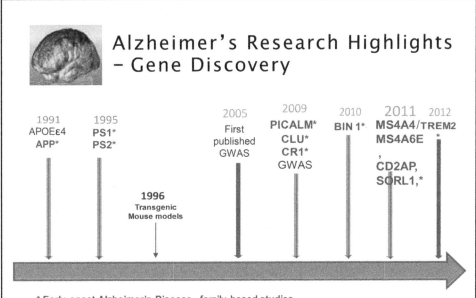

Fig. 12 (Illustration Courtesy of the National Institute on Aging, National Institutes of Health, U.S. Department of Health and Human Services)

Several other Alzheimer's genetic research initiatives—the Alzheimer's Disease Sequencing Project, the International Genomics of Alzheimer's Project, and the Alzheimer's Genome Project, seek to further build on GWAS to more precisely determine the role of newly discovered genes and their variants in Alzheimer's disease.

The future of LOAD prevention strategies will eventually include the evaluation of multiple sets of genes and their variants. The evaluation of an individual's polygenic architecture enables invaluable insights into a person's risk, and the opportunity to modify that risk beyond a **single nucleotide polymorphism** assessment of ApoE.

Single Nucleotide Polymorphism *(SNP-pronounced snip)— a sequence variation of a single DNA base (nucleotide). ApoE4 variant is determined by two SNPs on the ApoE gene.*

Polygenic risk/hazard scores are the subject of recent research efforts in "quantifying individual differences in age-specific risk of Alzheimer's disease". (83)

A recent study that utilized a validated polygenic hazard score that included 1,081 asymptomatic older adults "significantly predicted risk of progression to Alzheimer's, even for people who do not have ApoE4 and in the cognitively normal." (84)

Undoubtedly, the future of a Alzheimer's polygenic score analysis into a comprehensive risk assessment is promising.

For now, we have bountiful evidence to leverage genetic risk assessments in LOAD. The ApoE4 gene variant and other risk variants have a growing body of study that elucidates their combined role in the accumulation and clearance of beta-amyloid peptide aggregates. (85)

In addition, recent and promising research has uncovered gene-gene interactions between ApoE and several other risk genes and their respective variants.

The inclusion of genetic biomarkers for methylation, such as the MTHFR gene variant (previously described on pages 35-36), mitochondrial function and brain atrophy (TOMM40), neuroinflammation (TREM2), and other variants, to the known functional and structural vulnerabilities linked to the ApoE4 variant which includes:

- glucose hypometabolism,

- mitochondrial dysfunction,

- impaired cholesterol metabolism,

- chronic inflammation,

- increased beta-amyloid peptide deposition and reduced clearance, and

- reduced hippocampal volume and greater rates of brain and hippocampal atrophy,

can serve immensely in a comprehensive risk reduction and personalized medicine framework that includes the evaluation of environmental, dietary and lifestyle factors that directly impact these genetic associations and vulnerabilities in LOAD. (86,87,88,89,90,91)

The aforementioned genomic research initiatives will undoubtedly provide new opportunities to add to that objective and further the exciting and emerging field of **genomic medicine**.

Genomic medicine: *"an emerging medical discipline that involves using genomic information about an individual as part of their clinical care (e.g., for diagnostic or therapeutic decision-making) and the health outcomes and policy implications of that clinical use."**

* National Human Genome Research Institute

Beta-Amyloid Protein

The early stages in the progression of brain insulin resistance and loss of synaptic integrity in LOAD is marked by the increase of beta-amyloid peptide aggregates referred to as soluble beta-amyloid oligomers (see illustration on next page). Thus, genetic and molecular biomarker assessments that provide insights into the potential risk for beta-amyloid burdens are prime opportunities for risk reduction and early intervention strategies.

Beta-amyloid oligomers *are soluble and more easily dispersed throughout the brain. As beta-amyloid oligomers aggregate and accumulate, they form insoluble amyloid fibrils and plaque deposits.*

The processing, aggregation, and build up of beta-amyloid peptides cleaved from amyloid precursor protein and the subsequent deposition of these peptides as the main component of amyloid plaque has long been theorized to be the central process associated with the neuropathological features of Alzheimer's.

However, numerous studies seeking to define the essential nature of beta-amyloid protein in the pathogenesis of Alzheimer's have demonstrated that a precursor to insoluble amyloid plaques, amyloid-beta derived diffusible ligands (ADDLs) that are cleaved from amyloid precursor protein are more toxic than the amyloid plaques they eventually form and are largely responsible for the cognitive deficits that occur in Alzheimer's.(92)

The neurotoxic effect of ADDLs is decidedly upstream of the aggregation and deposition of insoluble amyloid plaque. ADDLs exert their damaging effects through several molecular mechanisms that results in the induction of oxidative stress and pro-inflammatory pathways, and the disruption of synaptic receptor mediated signaling cascades vital to synaptic plasticity. (93)

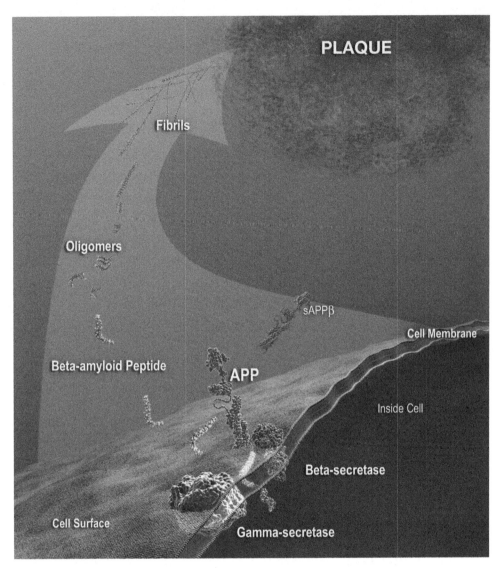

Fig. 13 (Illustration Courtesy of the National Institute on Aging, National Institutes of Health, U.S. Department of Health and Human Services)

Description of Fig. 13:

The first byproducts of amyloid precursor protein (APP) cleavage by enzymes (secretases) produces monomers of beta-amyloid peptide. These non-aggregated peptides eventually form assemblies into oligomers. A range of sizes and peptide conformations make up oligomeric assemblies, including ADDLs. In Alzheimer's these oligomeric aggregates form amyloid fibrils which deposit into amyloid plaques.

Research shows that levels of brain insulin receptors are lower in individuals with Alzheimer's disease. Underlying this insulin/Alzheimer's axis is the impact of ADDLs and their binding with insulin receptors at a crucial locus of memory and learning facilitation—the synapse.

This ADDL-mediated impairment of the insulin receptor and other synaptic receptors leads to the loss of synapse function vital to the connectivity between brain cells and a healthy brain that can learn and retain information.

Apart from the effect of ADDLs on synaptic receptors and function, ADDLs migrate into neurons and wreak havoc on mitochondrial function and destabilize tau protein tubules that result in neurofibrillary tangles—one of the two principal hallmark lesions evident in Alzheimer's disease (illustrated in Fig. 5 on page 45).

Tau protein is a key assembly piece in the cytoskeletal and conveyance network of the neuron's axon extension and the breakdown of this critical system results in the lack of essential working parts (e.g., mitochondria), the energy currency (ATP) and nutrients (e.g., proteins, lipids) needed at axon terminals to support and power synaptic activity.

The transport and recycling of these elements to and from the neuronal terminals via axon microtubules (see Fig. 14 on next page) is vital to the optimal functioning of the neuron and its synapses.(94)

The last few paragraphs and the illustration above are intended to highlight the damaging force that is initiated by beta-amyloid aggregates (ADDLs) upon mitochondrial function and the neuron's intricate orchestration of mitochondrial trafficking that is required for maintaining the high energy demands of the synapse and synaptic transmission.

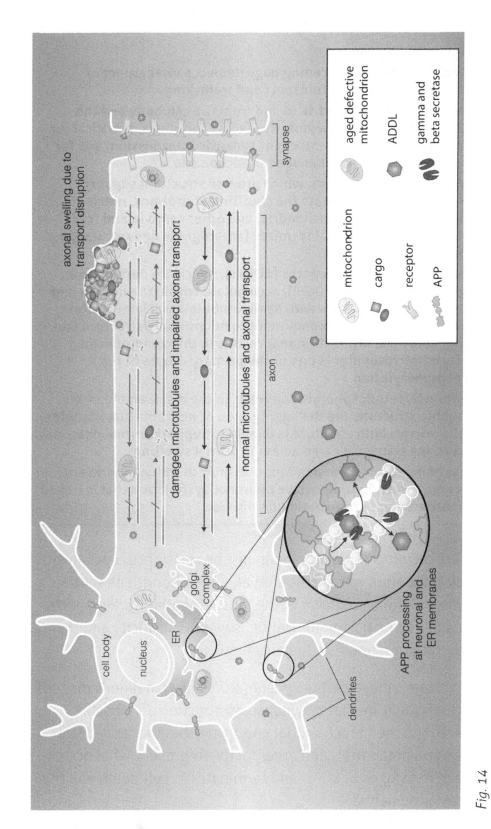

Fig. 14
See description of illustration on next page.

Description of Fig. 14:

The illustration on the preceding page depicts a vital aspect of neuronal function: axonal transport and trafficking.

The transport of mitochondria to and from the cell body and the endpoints of the neuron's axons, the axonal terminals, is critical for meeting the energy requirements of synaptic transmission, and for the recycling of worn and damaged mitochondria.

The microtubules of the axon which provide structural support are also the tracks that enable the shuttling of proteins, nutrients, organelles such as the mitochondria, and other cargo to and from the cell body and the axonal terminal (anterograde and retrograge transport).

Beta-amyloid protein aggregates (ADDLs), which are derived from amyloid precursor protein (APP), accumulate within the neuron and results in toxic interactions with a microtubule-associated protein, tau, which is an important component to microtubule structure and stability. This toxic interaction that results in the compromised integrity of microtubules is one of the primary causes of *tau hyperphosphorylation.*

Tau protein hyperphosphorylation leads to the disassembly of the microtubule structure and the aggregation of neurofibrillary tangles. Once the microtubule structure is unable to support normal neuronal transport, the transport cargo amass in axonal swellings.

The loss of microtubule-dependent transport of mitochondria and other cargo results in progressive neuronal dysfunction that is linked to the earliest stages of Alzheimer's disease.

ADDLs are an integral piece to brain insulin resistance mechanisms and their infiltration into the neuron and mitochondria is another component to the breakdown of the most essential working parts that enable neuronal communication, synaptic plasticity and the neuroenergetic engine that sustains it all.

To reemphasize, these pathological features of Alzheimer's disease that include ADDL mediated synapse dysfunction and insulin resistance, and the mitochondrial energy deficits that arise from glucose hypometabolism and other factors represent what occurs in the earliest stages of LOAD and terminates in cell death and the diagnosis of dementia.

With regard to insulin function, ADDLs effect neurological deficits by localizing at particular synapses and precipitating the loss of insulin receptor and synapse function. ADDLs are thought to prevent insulin receptors from accumulating at the synapse and effectively making them unable to respond to insulin and thus insulin resistant. (95) (See Fig. 15 on page 87). However, ADDL-mediated toxicity and disruption of signaling mechanisms at the synapse is not limited to insulin receptors only.

As essential as insulin and their associated receptors are in memory storage and retrieval, other synaptic receptors work in concert with insulin and the insulin receptor to effect a complex interaction of synaptic receptor mediated cascades that ultimately shape our cognitive coherence.(96)

The propensity of ADDLs to localize at the synapse, and at other sites on the neuron (extrasynaptic), impairs the functionality to several synaptic receptors (e.g., NMDAR, AMPAR, EphB2) that mediate signaling pathways which are critical in how learning and memory mechanisms are **soft-wired**. ADDLS ravage the synaptic terrain and thus are aptly described as "Synaptic Superdestroyers" of the brain.(97)

> **Soft-wired:** *the circuitry of our neural networks is not intrinsically fixed and hard-wired. The brain's soft-wired capacity to integrate and organize new information (neuroplasticiy—page 73) required in learning and memory processing reflects a malleable and dynamic brain that is able to grow (neurogenesis) and rewire it's vast neural connectivity.*

Excitotoxicity

The pathways of the signaling cascades facilitated by insulin and other stimuli (eg., glutamate) are enormously complex; therefore I will only briefly describe a key aspect that is central to neuroplasticity when all goes right, and how this pathway also represents a significant aspect of what can go wrong and greatly contribute to cognitive decline and LOAD. It centers on the regulation of calcium flux in the brain and is termed: "The Calcium Hypothesis of Brain Aging and Alzheimer's Disease" that was first proposed in 1983 and has since been the subject of many studies.

The calcium hypothesis of Alzheimer's postulates that the dysregulation of calcium homeostasis in the brain is a principal feature in the earliest pathological events of Alzheimer's and in the accelerated learning and memory impairment that occurs in the later stages and onset of Alzheimer's dementia. How does that work?

The N-methyl-D-aspartate receptor (NMDAR), and other synaptic receptors (e.g., AMPAR) are integral in the regulating the flux of calcium into the neuron.

Calcium functions as an integral signaling molecule in the brain and the regulated calcium flow through receptors and channels into the neuron triggers key signaling cascades that are central to brain plasticity.

Normal NMDAR excitability (response to an excitatory stimulus) and intracellular calcium messengering is an essential element in the cascade of mechanisms that potentiate learning, memory, and neuroplasticity.(98, 99) However, in Alzheimer's disease ADDLs promote cellular calcium overload by excessive activation of the NMDAR and family of associated receptors (glutamate receptors).

As with the insulin receptor, ADDLs bind to or in close proximity to the NMDAR—a glutamate receptor. (99) ADDLs induce dysfunction of NMDAR's role in calcium flux into the neuron through excessive activation (see Fig. 15 on next page).

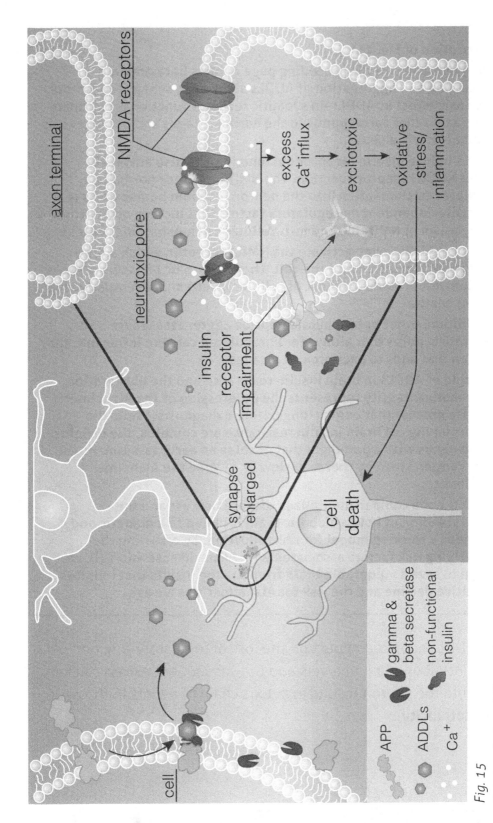

axon terminal

NMDA receptors

neurotoxic pore

insulin receptor impairment

excess Ca⁺ influx → excitotoxic → oxidative stress/ inflammation

synapse enlarged

cell death

cell

APP

gamma & beta secretase

ADDLs

non-functional insulin

Ca⁺

Fig. 15
See description of illustration on next page.

Description of Fig. 15:

The illustration on the preceding page depicts beta-amyloid processing and aggregation of ADDLs at, or near, synapse receptors. The toxic effect of ADDLs on synaptic receptor function is a primary component that corresponds to the earliest stages and pathogenesis of Alzheimer's disease.

ADDLs induce insulin receptor dysfunction and also adversely affect NMDA receptor function. The NMDA receptor normally regulates calcium influx into the neuron. Calcium homeostasis is normally dependent on regulatory factors that include magnesium antagonism of NMDARs, and intracellular calcium binding proteins.

However, ADDLs over-activate the NMDA receptor, which allows excess calcium influx into the cell. The excitotoxic effect from excess calcium influx leads to a host of cellular insults that eventually lead to cell death.

In addition, other beta-amyloid peptide aggregates create neurotoxic pores that allows for unregulated calcium influx into the neuron that adds to excitotoxic cascades.

The role of ADDLs in brain insulin resistance and the obliteration of synaptic integrity represents the progression of the Alzheimer's disease process that begins long before a diagnosis. While the underpinnings of brain insulin resistance are complex, the insights empower us with a paradigm that enables an early assessment and intervention strategy that may slow or reverse the Alzheimer's pandemic.

LOAD is not a compartmentalized disease process and the understanding of how a diabetic brain is linked to a diabetic body provides a working model for risk reduction. By arresting the underlying risk factors associated with heart disease and T2D, we begin to save a vulnerable brain from the the insults that initiates cognitive decline and the risk for Alzheimer's as we age.

The ADDL-mediated impact on the loss of regulatory function of the NMDAR on calcium levels and the subsequent excess calcium flow into the neuron results in a toxic chain of events in the neuron (**excitotoxicity**).

Excitotoxicity *is defined as the overstimulation or excessive exposure of glutamate receptors to the neurotransmitter glutamate or excitotoxins which impairs cellular calcium homeostasis, leading to neuronal injury or death.*

The excitotoxic cascades mediated by ADDLs and other insults on synaptic NMDARs are a major component to the synaptic degeneration and loss associated with Alzheimer's disease and many of these neurotoxic events occur unnoticed in the earliest stages of LOAD.

Chronic and moderate NMDAR activation by homocysteine and metabolic derivatives that include homocysteic acid are also potential inductors of NMDAR-mediated excitotoxicity.(100, 101)

Pro-inflammatory and oxidative stress patterns linked to neurofibrillary tangles and mitochondrial dysfunction contributes to glutamate receptor (NMDAR, AMPA) instability.

In aging, excessive glutamate release and the excitotoxic overactivation of glutamate receptors is further driven by impaired cerebral circulation and chronic brain ischemia (decreased blood flow to the brain) caused by atherosclerosis and cerebrovascular complications (transient ischemic attacks). In stroke, an acute and massive destabilization of glutamate levels occurs.

There is another collateral feature to the onslaught of excitotoxic injury in the brain. The cumulative load of calcium in the neuron results in blunted mitochondrial function and ATP metabolism (hypometabolism), and oxidative stress.(101)

Oxidative stress is a leading cause of oxidative damage in chronic brain ischemia and acute stroke. Stabilizing and optimizing mitochondrial function is critical to buffering and protecting against excitotoxic mechanisms that can overwhelm the neuron, and leads to oxidative DNA damage and cell death.

Antioxidants, botanical extracts (polyphenols), magnesium, taurine, ketone therapy, intermittent fasting, and caloric restriction are protective against calcium destabilization of the mitochondria and corrective in recovery from these excitotoxic insults.(102, 103, 104, 105, 106, 107)

Summary - In a Nutshell

To summarize, synaptic insulin function in the brain is a key element in memory, learning, and brain plasticity, and the disruption of that dynamic is central to the risk for cognitive impairment and for LOAD as we age.

The toxic ADDL disruption of insulin signaling and synaptic receptor function is central to the asymptomatic and earliest stages associated with LOAD and the progression to Alzheimer's dementia.

Sustained elevations of blood glucose and insulin, the peripheral insulin resistance that is associated with obesity, MetS, and T2D, and the associated complications of CVD, have profound effects on our brain and cognitive function as we age. The impairment of blood flow to the brain that is associated with these metabolic and vascular disorders adds another component of risk for vascular dementia and LOAD.

Oxidative stress and chronic inflammation in obesity, MetS, T2D, and CVD drives the molecular and biochemical cascades that further initiate pro-inflammatory and oxidative stress pathways in the brain.

A generally unrecognized risk factor in clinical practice is the integrity of mitochondrial function and energy metabolism in the brain that for vulnerable individuals predisposes them to oxidative stress and significant reductions in glucose metabolism, brain shrinkage, and gradual cognitive decline throughout a lifetime. Women are at increased risk.

In individuals with an increased genetic susceptibility to LOAD, these inherent predispositions and chronic age-related disease patterns result in the increased processing of beta-amyloid precursor protein and subsequent generation of ADDLs in the brain, which further precipitates brain insulin resistance, excitotoxic cascades, mitochondrial stress, disruptions in energy metabolism, tau protein aggregation and neurofibrillary tangles, and the eventual demise of the neuron.

These complex neurological perturbations of the diabetic brain do have a practical solution—prevention. We know that the risk for dementia is set in motion by a host of genetic and environmental risk factors that are pivotal at midlife. And we know that LOAD progresses over many years and that it is a silent disease in its preclinical stage years before there are any noticeable signs of cognitive impairment.

Throughout this book I have described the physiological roots of insulin resistance, T2D, and CVD that may easily mushroom into neurological disease later in life. We can be empowered by that understanding as it provides a roadmap for preemptive action—for taking control of the risk factors that may put our memories, our independence and our peace of mind at risk.

This awareness has led to a more enlightened Alzheimer's solution era ushered in by research and science that is advancing a personalized medicine approach (biomarker-guided medicine) to mitigate the growing health crisis of the Alzheimer's pandemic. "The Golden Gate for Detection, Treatment and Prevention of Alzheimer's Disease" is not just a futuristic goal. It stands in front of us as an accessible option.(108)

About the Author

Ralph Sanchez, MTCM, CNS, has authored two books, *The Diabetic Brain In Alzheimer's disease* and *The Improved MIND Diet*.

Ralph currently lives in Carmel, CA where he spends most of his time creating information based products that enable a deeper understanding for reducing the risk for Alzheimer's disease. His third book is in development.

Ralph's mission is: *"To enhance and build awareness on the Alzheimer's disease pandemic and the cutting edge science and resources that contributes to its reversal"*.

To find out more about Ralph and his personalized body-brain renewal program—BrainDefend™, please visit BrainDefend.com and TheAlzheimersSolution.com.

In Memoriam

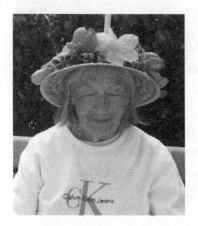

The photograph is my mother. It was taken by my sister on a Cinco de Mayo party a few years ago at the home where she resided. Mom passed away in July of 2016 from complications related to vascular dementia.

Mom's photograph seems to capture a moment of peace. My sister and I were blessed that Mom saved for this time of life and that she could be in a place where she was supervised, entertained, socially engaged, well fed, and kept safe. We were fortunate to have many other smiling moments of Mom photographed over her last few years.

However, I know in my heart that without the oversight that my sister provided and the input I was able to give with regard to nutritional needs, Mom would not have done as well as she did over her remaining years once it was decided that she no longer could live alone.

One of the most difficult challenges that arise in caring for aging individuals is the quality of support that is available. In dementia, that becomes a monumental concern as the affordability of quality assisted living centers for individuals with cognitive impairment or dementia is prohibitive.

This book is dedicated to my mother and all of the mothers and fathers who must be placed in elder care centers that specialize in providing the services and care needed for aging individuals in cognitive decline. May they all be as well provided for as they deserve.

Sincerely,

Ralph Sanchez

"The soundness of our mind is built on a plastic brain— malleable, adaptable and reinventing its form and function as needed. What nurtures it, or why it unravels in aging, is the key to an Alzheimer's solution."

~Ralph Sanchez

References

1. The Obesity, Metabolic Syndrome, and Type 2 Diabetes Mellitus Pandemic: Part I. Increased Cardiovascular Disease Risk and the Importance of Atherogenic Dyslipidemia in Persons With the Metabolic Syndrome and Type 2 Diabetes Mellitus

Henry N. Ginsberg, MD and Paul R. MacCallum, PhD

J Cardiometab Syndr. 2009 Spring; 4(2): 113–119.

2. Alzheimer's disease drug-development pipeline: few candidates, frequent failures

Jeffrey L Cummings, Travis Morstorf and Kate Zhong

Alzheimer's Research & Therapy 2014 July 3, 2014 6:37

3. Age and amyloid effects on human central nervous system amyloid-beta kinetics

Patterson BW, Elbert DL, Mawuenyega KG, et al.

Ann Neurol. 2015;78(3):439–453.

4. Shared genetic etiology underlying Alzheimer's disease and type 2 diabetes

Hao K, Di Narzo AF, Ho L, Luo W, Li S, Chen R, Li T, Dubner L, Pasinetti GM.

Mol Aspects Med. 2015 Jun-Oct;43-44:66-76.

5. Pathophysiologic relationship between Alzheimer's disease, cerebrovascular disease, and cardiovascular risk: A review and synthesis

Santos CY, Snyder PJ, Wu W-C, Zhang M, Echeverria A, Alber J.

Alzheimer's & Dementia : Diagnosis, Assessment & Disease Monitoring. 2017;7:69-87.

6. The metabolic syndrome and mortality from cardiovascular disease and all-causes: Findings from the National Health and Nutrition Examination Survey II Mortality Study

Ford ES

Atherosclerosis 173 : 309 –314, 2004.

7. Diagnosis and management of the metabolic syndrome: an American Heart Association/National Heart, Lung, and Blood Institute scientific statement: executive summary

Grundy SM, Cleeman JI, Daniels SR, Donato KA, Eckel RH, Franklin BA, Gordon DJ, Krauss RM, Savage PJ, Smith J

8. Metabolic syndrome–a new world-wide definition. A Consensus Statement from the International Diabetes Federation

Alberti, K. G., Zimmet, P. & Shaw, J.

Diabetic medicine: a journal of the British Diabetic Association 23, 469–480.

9. A Comprehensive Review on Metabolic Syndrome

Jaspinder Kaur

Cardiol Res Pract. 2014; 2014: 943162.

10. Centers for Disease Control and Prevention. National diabetes factsheet: national estimates and general information on diabetes and prediabetes in the United States, 2011

Atlanta, GA: US Department of Health and Human Services, Centers for Disease Control and Prevention, 2011.

11. Prediabetes: a high-risk state for diabetes development

Tabak AG, Herder C, Rathmann W, Brunner EJ, Kivimaki M.

Lancet. 2012;379:2279-90.

12. Linking type 2 diabetes and Alzheimer's disease

Weiping Hana, and Cai Li

PNAS April 13, 2010 vol. 107 no. 15 6557-6558

13. Increased risk of type 2 diabetes in Alzheimer disease

Janson J, Laedtke T, Parisi JE, O'Brien P, Petersen RC, Butler PC

Diabetes. 2004 Feb; 53(2):474-81.

14. Type 2 Diabetes as a Risk Factor for Dementia in Women Compared With Men: A Pooled Analysis of 2.3 Million People Comprising More Than 100,000 Cases of Dementia

Saion Chatterjee, et al.

Diabetes Care 2016 Feb; 39(2): 300-307.

15. Global Epidemiology of Dementia: Alzheimer's and Vascular Types

Liara Rizzi, Idiane Rosset, and Matheus Roriz-Cruz

BioMed Research International Volume 2014 (2014), Article ID 908915, 8 pages

16. The Obesity, Metabolic Syndrome, and Type 2 Diabetes Mellitus Pandemic: Part I. Increased Cardiovascular Disease Risk

and the Importance of Atherogenic Dyslipidemia in Persons With the Metabolic Syndrome and Type 2 Diabetes Mellitus

Ginsberg HN, MacCallum PR.

Journal of the Cardiometabolic Syndrome. 2009;4(2):113-119.

17. Metabolically healthy obesity': Origins and implications

Gerald V. Denisa,* and Martin S. Obin

Mol Aspects Med. 2013 Feb; 34(1): 59–70.

18. Is There a Paradox in Obesity?

Goyal A, Nimmakayala KR, Zonszein J.

Cardiology in Review. 2014;22(4):163-170.

19. Comorbidities of Diabetes and Hypertension: Mechanisms and Approach to Target Organ Protection

Amanda N. Long, DO and Samuel Dagogo-Jack, MD

J Clin Hypertens (Greenwich). 2011 Apr; 13(4): 244–251.

20. Heart disease and stroke statistics - 2016 update: a report from the American Heart Association Statistics Committee and Stroke Statistics Subcommittee

Mozaffarian D, Benjamin EJ, Go AS, Arnett DK, Blaha MJ, Cushman M,Das SR, de Ferranti S, Després, JP, Fullerton HJ, Howard VJ, HuffmanMD, Isasi CR, Jiménez MC, Judd SE, Kissela BM, et al.

Circulation December 16, 2015. 12.

21. Vascular risk factors, cognitive decline, and dementia

E Duron and Olivier Hanon

Vasc Health Risk Manag. 2008 Apr; 4(2): 363–381.

22. Cardiovascular Risk Factors Promote Brain Hypoperfusion Leading to Cognitive Decline and Dementia

Jack C. de la Torre

Cardiovascular Psychiatry and Neurology Volume 2012, Article ID 367516, 15 pages

23. MTHFR C677T mutation increased the risk of Ischemic Stroke, especially in large-artery atherosclerosis in adults: an updated meta-analysis from 38 researches

Cui T1.

Int J Neurosci. 2016;126(1):10-9.

24. Common folate gene variant, MTHFR C677T, is associated with brain structure in two independent cohorts of people with mild cognitive impairment.

Rajagopalan P, Jahanshad N, Stein JL, et al.

NeuroImage Clinical. 2012;1(1):179-187.

25. Hyperhomocysteinemia: Impact on Neurodegenerative Diseases

Meenakshi Sharma, Manisha Tiwari, Rakesh Kumar Tiwar

Basic & Clinical Pharmacology & Toxicology, 2015, 117, 287–296

26. Association of RFC1 A80G and MTHFR C677T polymorphisms with Alzheimer's disease.

Bi XH, Zhao HL, Zhang ZX, Zhang JW.

Neurobiol Aging. 2009 Oct;30(10):1601-7.

27. Genetic and Environmental Risk for Alzheimer's disease Consortium (GERAD1) (2016). A Validation Study of Vascular

Cognitive Impairment Genetics Meta-Analysis Findings in an Independent Collaborative Cohort.

Skrobot, O. A., McKnight, A. J., Passmore, P. A., Seripa, D., Mecocci, P., Panza, F.et al.

Journal of Alzheimer's Disease, 53(3), 981-989.

28. US Census Bureau brief on age and sex, issued May 2011. Age and Sex Composition: Census Briefs, 2010

Lindsay M. Howden and Julie A. Meyer

www.census.gov/prod/cen2010/briefs/c2010br-03.pdf.

29. Alzheimer's Association. 2018 Alzheimer's Disease Facts and Figures

Alzheimers Dement 2018;14(3):367-429.

30. Summary of the evidence on modifiable risk factors for cognitive decline and dementia: A population-based perspective

Matthew Baumgart, Heather M.Snyder, Maria C.Carrillo, SamFazio, Hye Kim, HarryJohns

Alzheimer's & Dementia. Volume 11, Issue 6, June 2015, Pages 718-726

31. Nutrition, Brain Aging, and Neurodegeneration

James Joseph, Greg Cole, Elizabeth Head, and Donald Ingram

The Journal of Neuroscience, October 14, 2009 • 29(41):12795–12801 • 12795

32. Nutrition and prevention of Alzheimer's dementia

Arun Swaminathan and Gregory A. Jicha

Frontiers in Aging Neuroscience. October 2014, Volume 6, Article 282

33. Nutraceuticals in cognitive impairment and Alzheimer's disease

P.Mecocci1, C.Tinarelli, R.J.Schulz and M.C.Polidori

Frontiers in Aging Neuroscience. June 2014, Volume 5, Article 147

34. Epigenetic nutraceutical diets in Alzheimer's disease

S. Davinelli, V. Calabrese, D. Zella, Giovanni Scapagnini

The journal of nutrition, health & aging. November 2014, Volume 18, Issue 9, pp 800–805

35. Oxysterols in the pathogenesis of major chronic diseases

Giuseppe Poli, Fiorella Biasi, Gabriella Leonarduzzi

Redox Biology. Volume 1, Issue 1, 2013, Pages 125-130

36. The Oxidative Stress Metabolite 4-Hydroxynonenal Promotes Alzheimer Protofibril Formation

Sarah J. Siegel, Jan Bieschke, Evan T. Powers, and Jeffery W. Kelly

Biochemistry 46, 6, 1503-1510

37. The Maillard hypothesis on aging: time to focus on DNA

Baynes JW.

Ann N Y Acad Sci. 2002 Apr;959:360-7

38. The role of advanced glycation end products in various types of neurodegenerative disease: a therapeutic approach

Salahuddin P, Rabbani G, Khan RH.

Cell Mol Biol Lett. 2014;19(3):407–437.

39. Role of Methylglyoxal in Alzheimer's Disease

Cristina Angeloni, Laura Zambonin, and Silvana Hrelia

BioMed Research International Volume 2014 (2014), Article ID 238485, 12 pages

40. Increased expression of the receptor for advanced glycation end products in neurons and astrocytes in a triple transgenic mouse model of Alzheimer's disease

Bo-Ryoung Choi, Woo-Hyun Cho, Jiyoung Kim, Hyong Joo Lee, ChiHye Chung, Won Kyung Jeon and Jung-Soo Han

Experimental & Molecular Medicine (2014) 46, e75

41. Oral glycotoxins are a modifiable cause of dementia and the metabolic syndrome in mice and humans

Weijing Cai, Jaime Uribarri, Li Zhu, Xue Chen, Shobha Swamy, Zhengshan Zhao, Fabrizio Grosjean, Calogera Simonaro, George A. Kuchel, Michal Schnaider-Beeri, Mark Woodward, Gary E. Striker, and Helen Vlassara

PNAS 2014 111 (13) 4940-4945; published ahead of print February 24, 2014

42. Current perspectives on the health risks associated with the consumption of advanced glycation end products: recommendations for dietary management

Sotiria Palimeri, Eleni Palioura, and Evanthia Diamanti-Kandarakis

Diabetes Metab Syndr Obes. 2015; 8: 415–426.

43. Nutrition and AGE-ing: Focusing on Alzheimer's Disease

Abate G, Marziano M, Rungratanawanich W, Memo M, Uberti D.

Oxidative Medicine and Cellular Longevity. 2017;2017:7039816.

44. Oxidative Stress and Inflammation in Heart Disease: Do Antioxidants Have a Role in Treatment and/or Prevention?

Fredric J. Pashkow

International Journal of Inflammation. Volume 2011 (2011), Article ID 514623, 9 pages

45. Lipoproteins and lipid peroxidation in Alzheimer's disease

Bassett CN, Montine TJ.

J Nutr Health Aging. 2003;7(1):24-9.

46. Evidence of increased oxidative damage in subjects with mild cognitive impairment

Keller JN, Schmitt FA, Scheff SW, Ding Q, Chen Q, Butterfield DA, Markesbery WR.

Neurology. 2005 Apr 12;64(7):1152-6.

47. Linking cardiometabolic disorders to sporadic ad: a perspective on potential mechanisms and mediators

Narayan R. Bhat

J Neurochem. Nov 2010; 115(3): 551–562.

48. Alzheimer Disease: Mercury as pathogenetic factor and apolipoprotein E as a moderator

Joachim Mutter, Johannes Naumann, Catharina Sadaghiani, Rainer Schneider & Harald Walach

Neuroendocrinology Letters No.5 October Vol.25, 2004

49. Methylmercury induces the expression of TNF- selectively in the brain of mice

Miyuki Iwai-Shimada, Tsutomu Takahashi, Min-Seok Kim, Masatake Fujimura, Hitoyasu Ito, Takashi Toyama, Akira Naganuma and Gi-Wook Hwang

Scientific Reports 6, Article number: 38294 (2016)

50. Pro-inflammatory gene expression and neurotoxic effects of activated microglia are attenuated by absence of CCAAT/ enhancer binding protein β

Marco Straccia, Núria Gresa-Arribas, Guido Dentesano, Aroa Ejarque-Ortiz, Josep M Tusell, Joan Serratosa, Carme Solà, and Josep Saura

Journal of Neuroinflammation 2011, 8:156

51. Shift in Brain Metabolism in Late Onset Alzheimer's Disease: Implications for Biomarkers and Therapeutic Interventions

Yao J, Rettberg JR, Klosinski LP, Cadenas E, Brinton RD.

Mol Aspects Med. 2011 August; 32(0): 247–257.

52. Insulin in Central Nervous System: More than Just a Peripheral Hormone

Ana I. Duarte, Paula I.Moreira, and Catarina R. Oliveira

Journal of Aging Research. Volume 2012, Article ID 384017, 21 pages

53. Lactate: the ultimate cerebral oxidative energy substrate?

Schurr A.

J Cereb Blood Flow Metab. 2006 Jan;26(1):142-52.

54. A cross-sectional comparison of brain glucose and ketone metabolism in cognitively healthy older adults, mild cognitive impairment and early Alzheimer's disease

E. Croteau, C.A. Castellano, M. Fortier, C. Bocti, T. Fulop, N. Paquet, S.C. Cunnane

Exp Gerontol. 2018 Jul 1;107:18-26.

55. Brain glucose hypometabolism and oxidative stress in preclinical Alzheimer's disease

Mosconi L, Pupi A, De Leon MJ.

Ann N Y Acad Sci. 2008 Dec;1147:180-95.

56. Functional brain abnormalities in young adults at genetic risk for late-onset Alzheimer's dementia

Reiman EM, Chen K, Alexander GE, Caselli RJ, Bandy D, Osborne D, Saunders AM, Hardy J.

Proc Natl Acad Sci U S A. 2004 Jan 6;101(1):284-9. Epub 2003 Dec 19.

57. Declining brain activity in cognitively normal apolipoprotein Eepsilon 4 heterozygotes: A foundation for using positron emission tomography to efficiently test treatments to prevent Alzheimer's disease

Reiman EM, Caselli RJ, Chen K, Alexander GE, Bandy D

Proc Natl Acad Sci U S A. 2001 Mar 13;98(6):3334-9.

58. Caloric restriction increases ketone bodies metabolism and preserves blood flow in aging brain

Lin A-L, Zhang W, Gao X, Watts L.

Neurobiology of Aging. 2015;36(7):2296-2303.

59. Fatty Acid-Binding Protein 5 Facilitates the Blood–Brain Barrier Transport of Docosahexaenoic Acid

Yijun Pan, Martin J. Scanlon, Yuji Owada, Yui Yamamoto§, Christopher J. H. Porter, and Joseph A. Nicolazzo

Mol. Pharmaceutics, 2015, 12 (12), pp 4375–4385

60. Medium-chain fatty acids inhibit mitochondrial metabolism in astrocytes promoting astrocyte-neuron lactate and ketone body shuttle systems

Thevenet J, De Marchi U, Domingo JS, Christinat N, Bultot L, Lefebvre G, Sakamoto K, Descombes P, Masoodi M, Wiederkehr A.

FASEB J. 2016 May; 30(5):1913-26.

61. Energy Contribution of Octanoate to Intact Rat Brain Metabolism Measured by 13C Nuclear Magnetic Resonance Spectroscopy

Douglas Ebert, Ronald G. Haller and Marlei E. Walton

The Journal of Neuroscience, July 2, 2003 • 23(13):5928 –5935

62. Fatty Acids in Energy Metabolism of the Central Nervous System

Alexander Panov, Zulfiya Orynbayeva, Valentin Vavilin, and Vyacheslav Lyakhovich

BioMed Research International. Volume 2014, Article ID 472459, 22 pages

63. Mechanisms of action for the medium-chain triglyceride ketogenic diet in neurological and metabolic disorders

Katrin Augustin, Aziza Khabbush, Sophie Williams, Simon Eaton, Michael Orford, J Helen Cross, Simon J R Heales, Matthew C Walker, Robin S B Williams

The Lancet Neurology. January 2018, Vol 17

64. Early Decline in Glucose Transport and Metabolism Precedes Shift to Ketogenic System in Female Aging and Alzheimer's Mouse Brain: Implication for Bioenergetic Intervention

Fan Ding, Jia Yao, Jamaica R. Rettberg, Shuhua Chen, Roberta Diaz Brinton

PLoS ONE 8(11): e79977.

65. Dietary ketosis enhances memory in mild cognitive impairment

Robert Krikoriana,*, Marcelle D Shidlera, Krista Dangelob, Sarah C Couchb, Stephen C Benoita, and Deborah J Clegg

Neurobiol Aging. 2012 February; 33(2): 425.e19–425.e27.

66. Ketogenic diets and Alzheimer's disease

Klaus W. Langea, Katharina M. Lange, Ewelina Makulska-Gertruda, Yukiko Nakamura, Andreas Reissmann, Shigehiko Kanaya, Joachim Hauser

Food Science and Human Wellness 6 (2017) 1–9

67. Effects of ketone bodies in Alzheimer's disease in relation to neural hypometabolism, β-amyloid toxicity, and astrocyte function

Hertz, L., Chen, Y. and Waagepetersen, H. S. (2015)

J. Neurochem., 2015, 134: 7–20.

68. Regulation of mitochondrial biogenesis

François R. Jornayvaz* and Gerald I. Shulman

Essays Biochem. 2010; 47:

69. The neuroprotective properties of calorie restriction, the ketogenic diet, and ketone bodies

Maalouf MA, Rho JM, Mattson MP.

Brain Research Reviews. 2009;59(2):293-315.

70. A low-carbohydrate, ketogenic diet to treat type 2 diabetes

Yancy WS, Foy M, Chalecki AM, Vernon MC, Westman EC.

Nutrition & Metabolism. 2005;2:34.

71. A Novel Intervention Including Individualized Nutritional Recommendations Reduces Hemoglobin A1c Level, Medication Use, and Weight in Type 2 Diabetes

McKenzie AL, Hallberg SJ, Creighton BC, Volk BM, Link TM, Abner MK, Glon RM, McCarter JP, Volek JS, Phinney SD

JMIR Diabetes 2017;2(1):e5

72. Long-term effects of a ketogenic diet in obese patients

Dashti HM, Mathew TC, Hussein T, et al.

Experimental & Clinical Cardiology. 2004;9(3):200-205.

73. Can Ketones Help Rescue Brain Fuel Supply in Later Life? Implications for Cognitive Health during Aging and the Treatment of Alzheimer's Disease.

Cunnane SC, Courchesne-Loyer A, Vandenberghe C, et al.

Frontiers in Molecular Neuroscience. 2016;9:53.

74. Maternal family history is associated with Alzheimer's disease biomarkers

Honea RA, Vidoni ED, Swerdlow RH, Burns JM; Alzheimer's Disease Neuroimaging Initiative.

J Alzheimers Dis. 2012;31(3):659-68.

75. Hypometabolism as a therapeutic target in Alzheimer's disease

Lauren C Costantini, Linda J Barr, Janet L Vogel and Samuel T Henderson

BMC Neuroscience 2008, 9(Suppl 2):S16

76. A new way to produce hyperketonemia: use of ketone ester in a case of Alzheimer's

Newport MT, VanItallie TB, Kashiwaya Y, King MT, Veech RL.

Alzheimer's & dementia: The Journal of the Alzheimer's Association. 2015;11(1):99-103.

77. White Matter Lipids as a Ketogenic Fuel Supply in Aging Female Brain: Implications for Alzheimer's Disease

Lauren P. Klosinski, Jia Yao, Fei Yin, Alfred N. Fonteh, Michael G. Harrington, Trace A. Christensen, Eugenia Trushina, Roberta Diaz Brinton

EBioMedicine 2 (2015) 1888–1904

78. Alzheimer's Association. 2016 Alzheimer's Disease Facts and Figures

Alzheimer's & Dementia 2016;12(4).

79. Insulin receptor signaling in the development of neuronal structure and function

Shu-Ling Chiu and Hollis T

Neural Development 2010 5:7

80. Role of insulin and insulin receptor in learning and memory

Zhao WQ, Alkon DL.

Mol Cell Endocrinol. 2001 May 25;177(1-2):125-34.

81. Shared Genetic Etiology between Type 2 Diabetes and Alzheimer's Disease Identified by Bioinformatics Analysis

Gao L, Cui Z, Shen L, Ji HF.

J Alzheimers Dis. 2016;50(1):13-7.

82. Pathophysiologic relationship between Alzheimer's disease, cerebrovascular disease, and cardiovascular risk: A review and synthesis

Santos CY, Snyder PJ, Wu W-C, Zhang M, Echeverria A, Alber J.

Alzheimer's & Dementia : Diagnosis, Assessment & Disease Monitoring. 2017;7:69-87.

83. Genetic assessment of age-associated Alzheimer disease risk: Development and validation of a polygenic hazard score

Desikan RS, Fan CC, Wang Y, Schork AJ, Cabral HJ, et al.

PLoS Med (2017) 14(3): e1002258.

84. Polygenic hazard scores in preclinical Alzheimer disease

Tan CH, Hyman BT, Tan JJX, Hess CP, Dillon W1, Schellenberg GD, et al.

Ann Neurol. 2017 Sep;82(3):484-488.

85. TREM2 Binds to Apolipoproteins, Including APOE and CLU/ APOJ, and Thereby Facilitates Uptake of Amyloid-Beta by Microglia

Yeh, Felix L. et al.

Neuron, Volume 91, Issue 2, 328-340

86. TREM2 upregulation correlates with 5-hydroxymethycytosine enrichment in Alzheimer's disease hippocampus

Celarain N, Sánchez-Ruiz de Gordoa J, Zelaya MV, et al.

Clinical Epigenetics. 2016;8:37.

87. Global changes in DNA methylation and hydroxymethylation in Alzheimer's disease human brain

Coppieters, Natacha et al.

Neurobiology of Aging, Volume 35, Issue 6, 1334 - 1344

88. APOE genotype and stress response -a mini review

Dose et al.

Lipids in Health and Disease (2016) 15:121

89. APOE Modulates the Correlation Between Triglycerides, Cholesterol, and CHD Through Pleiotropy, and Gene-by-Gene Interactions

Taylor J. Maxwell, Christie M. Ballantyne, James M. Cheverud, Cameron S. Guild, Chiadi E. Ndumele and Eric Boerwinkle

GENETICS December 1, 2013 vol. 195 no. 4 1397-1405;

90. Association of Chronic Low-grade Inflammation With Risk of Alzheimer Disease in ApoE4 Carriers

Tao Q, Ang TFA, DeCarli C, et al.

JAMA Netw Open. 2018;1(6):e183597.

91. Synergistic interaction between APOE and family history of Alzheimer's disease on cerebral amyloid deposition and glucose metabolism

Dahyun Yi, Younghwa Lee, Min Soo Byun, Jun Ho Lee, Kang Ko, Bo Kyung Sohn, Young Min Choe, Hyo Jung Choi, Hyewon Baek, Chul-Ho Sohn, Yu Kyeong Kim, Dong Young Lee

Alzheimer's Research & Therapy. 2018, 10:84

92. Molecular mechanisms of amyloid oligomers toxicity

Kayed R, Lasagna-Reeves CA

J Alzheimers Dis. 2013;33 Suppl 1:S67-78.

93. Alzheimer's disease, beta-amyloid, glutamate, NMDA receptors and memantine – searching for the connections

Wojciech Danysz and Chris G Parsons Br

J Pharmacol. 2012 September; 167(2): 324–352.

94. Abnormal tau, mitochondrial dysfunction, impaired axonal transport of mitochondria, and synaptic deprivation in Alzheimer's disease

P. Hemachandra Reddy

Brain Res. 2011 September 30; 1415: 136–148.

95. Amyloid beta oligomers induce impairment of neuronal insulin receptors

Wei-Qin Zhao, Fernanda G. De Felice, Sara Fernandez, et al.

FASEB J. 2008 Jan;22(1):246-60. Epub 2007 Aug 24.

96. Insulin promotes rapid delivery of N-methyl-d- aspartate receptors to the cell surface by exocytosis

Vytenis A. Skeberdis, Jian-yu Lan, Xin Zheng, R. Suzanne Zukin, and Michael V. L. Bennett

PNAS March 13, 2001 98 (6) 3561-356

97. Mechanisms of synapse and dendrite maintenance and their disruption in psychiatric and neurodegenerative disorders

Lin YC, Koleske AJ.

Annu Rev Neurosci. 2010;33:349–378.

98. Activation Mechanisms of the NMDA Receptor

Blanke ML, VanDongen AMJ

SourceBiology of the NMDA Receptor. Boca Raton (FL): CRC Press; 2009. Chapter 13. Frontiers in Neuroscience

99. Abeta oligomers induce neuronal oxidative stress through an N-methyl-D-aspartate receptor-dependent mechanism that is blocked by the Alzheimer drug memantine

De Felice, F. G., Velasco, P. T., Lambert, M. P., Viola, K., Fernandez, S. J., Ferreira, S. T., Klein, W. L.

J. Biol. Chem. 282, 11590-11601, (2007)

100. Chemical Pathology of Homocysteine. IV. Excitotoxicity, Oxidative Stress, Endothelial Dysfunction, and Inflammation

Kilmer S. McCully

Ann Clin Lab Sci Summer 2009 vol. 39 no. 3 219-232

101. Treatment of Alzheimer's Disease with Anti-Homocysteic Acid Antibody in 3xTg-AD Male Mice

Hasegawa T, Mikoda N, Kitazawa M, LaFerla FM

PLoS ONE, 2010 5(1): e8593.

102. Oxidative Stress and the Use of Antioxidants in Stroke

Shirley R, Ord EN, Work LM.

Antioxidants (Basel). 2014;3(3):472–501. Published 2014 Jul 3.

103. Herbal Medicine: Biomolecular and Clinical Aspects. 2nd edition

Albert Y. Sun, Qun Wang, Agnes Simonyi, and Grace Y. Sun

Chapter 15: Botanical Phenolics and Neurodegeneration

104. Nutrition and Traumatic Brain Injury: Improving Acute and Subacute Health Outcomes in Military Personnel (2011)

Chapter: 14 Polyphenols

105. Magnesium Sulfate Protects Against the Bioenergetic Consequences of Chronic Glutamate Receptor Stimulation

Pascaline Clerc, Christina A. Young, Evan A. Bordt, Alina M. Grigore, Gary Fiskum, Brian M. Polster

PLoS ONE 8(11): e79982.

106. Ketones inhibit mitochondrial production of reactive oxygen species production following glutamate excitotoxicity by increasing NADH oxidation.

Maalouf M, Sullivan PG, Davis L, Kim DY, Rho JM.

Neuroscience. 2007;145(1):256–264.

107. Caloric restriction increases brain mitochondrial calcium retention capacity and protects against excitotoxicity

Ignacio Amigo, Sergio Luiz Menezes Filho, Luis Alberto Luévano Martínez, Bruno Chausse, Alicia J. Kowaltowski

Aging Cell(2017)16, pp73–81

108. Precision Medicine - The Golden Gate for Detection, Treatment and Prevention of Alzheimer's Disease

Hampel H, O'Bryant SE, Castrillo JI, et al.

The Journal of Prevention of Alzheimer's disease. 2016;3(4):243-259.

Notes

Notes

Notes

Notes

Notes

Made in the USA
Las Vegas, NV
04 April 2024

88264317R00070